PRAISE FOR DEPRE
DARKNESS ANL

MW00399365

In this courageous and powerful book, Dr. Dan Hale provides insightful perspectives on depression from his own personal struggles with the illness, his experiences as the father of a daughter who battled and eventually lost her fight with it, and his insights gained as a psychologist as well as a person of faith. Stories containing raw emotions, honest self-examination, and a deep search for understanding and healing, will leave readers — whether they suffer from depression themselves, deal with it as health professionals or faith leaders, live with others who have it, or know others who do — well informed, inspired to seek help, engage in self-care, remain hopeful, and reach out to those who have suffered in the shadows for so long from this crippling illness. I am so grateful for Dr. Hale's courage in bringing his stories of depression out of the darkness into the light – where we can, if we commit to doing the same, restore healing and hope for generations to come.

—Lisa A. Cooper, MD, MPH, FACP
Bloomberg Distinguished Professor
James F. Fries Professor of Medicine
Johns Hopkins University School of Medicine, School of
Nursing, and Bloomberg School of Public Health

In Depression — Out of the Darkness and Into the Light, Dr. Dan Hale provides an invaluable resource for individuals, families, friends, congregations and communities who seek to educate themselves about signs and symptoms of this serious mental illness, as well as successful treatment options, and resources for fostering resilience and hope. As a psychologist and professor, Dr. Hale is well-positioned to speak about this illness from a clinical perspective; however, what makes this book such an important and welcome addition to literature in this field is his candor in sharing both his personal experience of living with major depression himself and his experiences parenting a child whose long struggle with depression eventually led to death by suicide. Dr. Hale accomplishes so much in this brief, powerful book: raising awareness about this potentially fatal mental illness, combating the pervasive stigma that too often prevents people from seeking help, equipping individuals and communities with concrete action items they can take to care for themselves and loved ones who struggle with depression, and offering personal testimony and clinically-based reassurance that there is indeed a path out of the darkness and into the light.

—The Rev. Kate Dunn
Associate Pastor for Congregational Care and Outreach
Fifth Avenue Presbyterian Church, New York, New York

Dr. Hale's book, Depression – Out of the Darkness and Into the Light, will capture the hearts, minds and spirits of those who suffer with depression and the family members and friends who care for them. By being transparent and vulnerable as he writes about his personal struggles with depression and the many difficult challenges he experienced caring for a daughter who eventually lost her life to this terrible illness, he opens a new avenue for people to understand and speak more freely about similar experiences. Readers will leave feeling a sense of camaraderie with the author. This book also can serve as a valuable resource for clergy and laity who feel called to minister to those impacted by depression.

—The Rev. Debra Hickman
Co-Founder/CEO of Sisters Together And Reaching (STAR)
Baltimore, Maryland

Any number of books on depression are available for the interested reader. However, many are dry and technical. This book, Depression – Out of the Darkness and Into the Light, is quite different. It is a powerful and personal story about one man's journey through bouts of depression and the suicide of his daughter. His experiences are vivid and poignant; he urges folks to talk openly about depression. Readers will find a deep and abiding understanding of disordered moods and thoughts in his eminently readable and clear insights. At the same time, the book offers descriptions of depression, its symptoms and treatment. It will appeal to family members and friends of a depressed person who are anxious to know how they may be of help. With its extensive list of resources to combat depression, it will be especially useful to members of faith communities and other institutions that can mobilize their members to recognize and be supportive of their depressed colleagues.

—Bonnie R. Strickland, PhD.
Professor of Psychology Emerita, University
of Massachusetts Amherst
Former President, American Psychological Association

Dr. Hale's book is grounded by professional training, but is profoundly accessible, personal, and readable through his stories. Although he is a trained psychologist, the author does not stand on a ledge of professional language as if he's looking at someone in a pit. Instead, he not only shares his own personal experience with depression and his experience regarding a beloved daughter with depression, we are invited to journey with him. We hear his own times of anguish and come out on the other side with concrete recommendations for treatments and support systems. In this meaningful work, readers learn the author's personal impetus for writing and then learn answers to many questions regarding the shadow of clinical depression. It is a complicated and elusive condition. Dr. Hale was especially helpful in describing the distorted worldview that depressed persons exhibit. Open this book and instantly be drawn into the stories and the descriptions — some raw and some gentle — regarding the conditions and treatments of clinical depression. This book is well worth the read.

—The Rev. Dr. Jeffrey Sumner
Senior Pastor, Westminster By-The-Sea Presbyterian Church
Daytona Beach Shores, Florida

Dan Hale has written a book that is extremely readable, but chock-full of excellent advice and information for anyone living with depression or anyone who cares about a family member, friend, or colleague living with depression. It is also an important book for faith communities as they seek to find ways to support congregants with depression and to educate others on ways to help. By intertwining the personal story of how depression impacted him, as well as the tragic loss of his daughter to the disease, Dr. Hale speaks with authenticity as a mental health clinician, a respected educator, and a loving father. His is a story that begs to be shared.

—Sherry Welch
Former Executive Director, NAMI Metropolitan Baltimore

Dr. Hale pulls back the curtain for his readers and allows them in the painful places of his life. He is transparent in the telling of his personal depressive episodes and he shares with a father's heart the sad story of his daughter's depression and the pain that came when the illness ultimately took her life. This book is an inspirational and faithful account of a family's walk through the dark valley of depression. It removes the mysteries associated with depression and reveals it for the ugly and sometimes dangerous monster that it is. In this book, the reader can find tools to assist them in recognizing the symptoms of depression, direction in finding the right mental health professionals to help one navigate the complexities of the illness, and hope for the recovery process. The book is written in a clear and easy-to-understand way and will be a good read for lay persons and professionals alike. I applaud Dr. Hale for his ability in blending his father's heart and his professional knowledge together to bring the subject of depression out of the darkness and into the light.

—The Rev. Pamula Yerby-Hammack
Assistant Pastor,
City of Abraham Church and Ministries
Baltimore, Maryland

Depression

Depression

*Out of the Darkness
and Into the Light*

W. DANIEL HALE, PhD

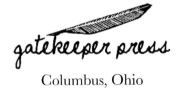

Columbus, Ohio

Depression - Out of the Darkness and Into the Light
Published by Gatekeeper Press
2167 Stringtown Rd, Suite 109
Columbus, OH 43123-2989
www.GatekeeperPress.com

ISBN (paperback): 9781642375756
eISBN: 9781642374711

Other Books by W. Daniel Hale

Building Healthy Communities Through
Medical-Religious Partnerships
with Richard G. Bennett and Panagis Galiatsatos

Healing Bodies and Souls: A Practical Guide for Congregations
with Harold G. Koenig

To Libby

CONTENTS

INTRODUCTION

Nothing could have prepared me for the brief talk I was to give that January evening at the church where my family and I had worshipped for more than three decades. Not my years of lecturing to college classes. Not my many presentations at professional conferences and community forums. This was a talk I had never given before — and one that every parent hopes they never have to give.

I was there to offer reflections on the life and death of my 36-year-old daughter, Libby, who had passed away just a few days before. As I prepared my remarks, Libby's sister and brother offered valuable guidance. They encouraged me to speak openly about the illness responsible for her death. If she had died of cancer, they noted, we would not be reluctant at all to talk about her battles and eventual death from it. But it was not cancer that took Libby from us. It was another terrible disease — depression.

Depression was not unfamiliar to me. I am a clinical psychologist and have devoted much of my research and clinical work to mood disorders. And I've also had personal experience with depression, having had two serious episodes that required medical and psychological treatment.

As I looked out at hundreds of people attending the memorial service that evening, I didn't know what type of response I would get to my remarks about Libby's struggles with depression and how she had taken her own life. But I felt strongly that I owed it to Libby and to all those still suffering with depression to use this dark moment in my life to shed light on this crippling and often lethal illness.

I must confess that I was surprised by just how many people spoke to my children and me after the service to express appreciation for my remarks – their words spoken with sincerity and purpose. The refrain, "We need to talk about depression," was repeated over and over again in these conversations. "We need to talk about depression in our schools." "We need to talk about depression in the workplace." "We need to talk about depression in our homes." "We need to talk about it in our churches."

I was truly touched by these comments, and especially moved over the next few weeks when I learned that many of these concerned individuals made generous donations to support the production of an educational video on depression that we chose to title, "We Need to Talk: A Story of Loss and Hope."

Since Libby's death, I have had many opportunities to share this video and to speak about depression in educational institutions, workplaces and religious congregations. Because of my longstanding interest in the intersection of faith and health, I was especially pleased to be invited to present at programs offered in faith communities. These programs were always well attended, and the audiences were always highly engaged. People came to learn, but they also came to share. They often talked about their own struggles with depression and how it had impacted their work, their relationships and even their faith. They spoke of periods when they felt completely worthless and helpless. They shared how, during these times, nothing in their life brought them any joy and how they could not imagine ever feeling hopeful about life again. Some even confessed to thinking at times about taking their own life. And many mentioned how this was the first time they had spoken openly to anyone about their depression.

The questions they asked also reflected a high degree of interest and concern. When does depression become so serious that it requires professional care? How does depression differ from grief? From stress? What treatments are available for depression?

Others who attended these programs came because they wanted to learn how to help a family member or friend who might be depressed. Sometimes the first thing they wanted to know was how to tell if a person is seriously depressed. What should they be looking for? Some wanted advice on how they could encourage their loved one to seek treatment. Besides helping them get professional care, what could they say and do to support them during the depths of their depression, before treatment takes effect? And many were concerned about the stress and strain they felt caring for someone who is depressed. What could they do so that their loved one's depression didn't drag them down into their own depression?

I also found it gratifying that at many of these programs there were individuals who were there not because they suffered from depression or had a loved one who did, but because they felt it was important for their congregation to minister to individuals and families affected by depression. What were some of the special challenges religious congregations might face as they try to identify and reach out to individuals who might be depressed? What could they do to erase the stigma that still is often associated with depression and that can serve as a barrier to seeking treatment? How could both clergy and laity reach out and support families who have lost a loved one to suicide?

As I gave these presentations, I learned how valuable it was for me to speak not only as a psychologist but also as someone who has suffered from depression and is willing to talk candidly about my own experiences. Again and again, I heard that talking about my own symptoms gave people a clearer and more in-depth understanding of what depression looked and felt like. But I found that there were other benefits to being open about my experience. People commented on how encouraging it was to hear someone speak about their own experiences with depression without any sense of shame or embarrassment. And they also spoke of how heartening it was to see someone who had been seriously depressed recover from the illness and return to an active life, full of love, joy and hope.

I also found that there was an appreciation for my willingness to speak from the heart about my daughter's struggles with depression and the many challenges family members faced as we tried to help Libby get the care and support she needed.

It was because of what I heard in these gatherings and in numerous conversations I have had with both clergy and concerned members of faith communities that I felt called to write *Depression – Out of the Darkness and Into the Light*. I heard repeatedly that there is a need in congregations in every community for more information about depression. There are people of faith struggling with depression who need to know that they are not alone and that there is hope. They need to know that their illness

> **There are people of faith struggling with depression who need to know that they are not alone and that there is hope.**

is not the result of a lack of faith or personal weakness. They need trustworthy information about the steps they can take to help them climb out of the dark depths of depression and into the light. And there are those who have loved ones suffering from depression and who need guidance about what they can say and do to be of help, and how to take care of themselves as they support their loved one.

There is also a need among concerned clergy and laity for information about how to minister to individuals and families affected by depression, in their congregations and their communities. What materials and resources are available? How can they work with health professionals in the community? How can they improve access to mental health services? These are the questions and concerns that guided me as I prepared *Depression – Out of the Darkness and Into the Light*.

W. DANIEL HALE, PhD

Chapter 1
A PERSONAL PERSPECTIVE

In this chapter, I offer an inside look at major depression, sharing what it was like for me – the overwhelming sadness, the loss of interest in things that had always brought me great joy, the terrible sleepless nights, the loss of my appetite, the constant state of exhaustion, the sense of worthlessness, the difficulty concentrating, the thoughts of death I could not get out of my mind, and a persistent sense of hopelessness. For those who have experienced depression, much of this should be familiar. For those who have not ever been depressed, this should give you a better idea of the devastating impact depression can have on almost every aspect of a person's life.

Chapter 2
A PROFESSIONAL'S PERSPECTIVE

I'm often asked why I have focused on depression for most of my career. Occasionally, a person will add, "Isn't it depressing to work with individuals suffering from depression?" In this chapter, I explain why I was drawn to depression at the beginning of my career and why, after more than forty years, I still find the work so rewarding and uplifting. I also share some of the encouraging lessons I have learned about depression, first as a psychotherapist and then later working with religious congregations to provide individuals suffering from depression with the information they need to recognize their condition, overcome any sense of embarrassment or shame about their illness, and seek professional care and the support of family and friends.

Chapter 3
A FATHER'S PERSPECTIVE

By the time Libby, our oldest child, reached the age of ten, she had established herself as one of the fastest young swimmers in the country. It wasn't unrealistic to think that someday she might swim in the Olympics. Like many of the girls she competed with who eventually became Olympians, Libby had the determination, drive and discipline it takes to succeed. But Libby's teenage years brought new challenges that derailed those ambitions. The most serious challenge came when she experienced the first of what would turn out to be several episodes of depression. Although she would recover from this initial episode, later episodes would prove to be more severe. It was during these later episodes that I experienced the painful frustration I had heard other parents talk about when they saw their adult children struggling with depression and other mental illnesses. You want to rush in and do everything you can to help them and to make sure they get the best possible care, but often you encounter limitations and obstacles you didn't have when they were younger and living under your roof. In this chapter, I discuss our efforts – some successful and others unsuccessful – to help Libby receive the care and support she needed and the lessons we learned from those experiences.

Chapter 4
RECOGNIZING AND RESPONDING TO DEPRESSION

While it is clear that depression is a painful and potentially lethal illness, there also is good news that needs to be shared – it is a highly treatable condition. However, far too many people who suffer from depression fail to receive effective treatment. One of the most common reasons is because individuals fail to recognize they are depressed. They may know that something is wrong, but they don't realize that what they are going through is a serious illness. In this chapter, I review the most common symptoms of depression and discuss how a diagnosis is made. After addressing additional barriers to treatment, I review treatment strategies and options, including the two most common approaches -- antidepressant medication and psychotherapy. I also share my own experiences working with my family physician, psychiatrist and psychologist during my two depressive episodes.

Chapter 5
CARING FOR A LOVED ONE

Caring for a loved one who is depressed can be challenging. You may find yourself experiencing confusion, frustration and a sense of helplessness. Some of the things depressed individuals say and do can be difficult to understand, and even hurtful. Because depression can have a serious, far-reaching impact on a person's attitudes, thoughts and behaviors, it's important for family members and friends to educate themselves as much as they can about this condition. In this chapter, I discuss how they can help their loved one receive the care, encouragement and support they need; how to recognize and respond to the risk of suicide; and the importance of self-care. I also share some examples of the valuable guidance, encouragement and support I received from family and friends during my darkest times.

Chapter 6
MINISTERING TO THE VULNERABLE AMONG US

One of the principal teachings of my faith is our responsibility to care for the most vulnerable among us. Growing up, the focus on caring for the vulnerable and suffering always meant reaching beyond the walls of the church. It didn't occur to me to also look inside the church. It wasn't until I began working with the seriously depressed that I realized many of the individuals experiencing the greatest sense of vulnerability and despair are sitting in our church pews on Sunday mornings, suffering in silence. In this chapter, I discuss how we can work toward creating communities where individuals experiencing the crippling pain and despair of depression can feel safe turning to their clergy and fellow congregants, confident they will receive the understanding, guidance and support they need.

Chapter 7
RESOURCES

Individuals experiencing depression, those who have a loved one suffering from depression and members of faith communities interested in ministering to those impacted by depression will find a wealth of resources in this chapter. Listed are organizations that offer online tools, fact sheets, brochures, classes, support groups and crisis services.

CHAPTER 1

A Personal Perspective

"I am truly blessed!" That is exactly what I thought — and often what I said out loud to myself — almost every day for the first 38 years of my life. Whether it was a weekday or the weekend, I knew my day would include a number of activities that I would thoroughly enjoy. This was especially true once I completed my training as a clinical psychologist and landed my dream job as a professor at Stetson University. I loved going to campus every day where I had the opportunity to work with bright, energetic students who were eager to learn about psychology and to use that knowledge to help others. And I was fortunate to have exceptional colleagues who provided plenty of intellectual stimulation and who were always there to support me, both professionally and personally.

Even during the most stressful periods in my life, I knew I could find pleasure in at least some of my daily endeavors. And I certainly could count on enjoying my time with family and friends. But all that changed dramatically when I found myself spiraling down into a deep, dark depression following a painful divorce. I had experienced periods of sadness before, but this was entirely different. I found that I no longer enjoyed being in the classroom, even when I was teaching my favorite courses. Nor did I enjoy meeting individually with students as they discussed their course projects or explored career options or shared exciting personal accomplishments. Conversations with colleagues over lunch or coffee had lost their appeal, as had weekly volleyball games with the other professors. To put it simply, I had lost interest in all aspects of my work life that previously had been so appealing and gratifying.

My inability to find any joy in activities that had previously brought me such great pleasure and a sense of fulfillment extended to my home life. I certainly didn't love my wonderful children – Libby (age 12), Graham (10) and Will (6) – any less, and I never forgot for even a moment how fortunate I was to have these three amazing children. I just couldn't enjoy my time with them the way that I had before. The things we had always liked doing together – taking bike rides, tossing a Frisbee, shooting baskets or just watching television – were no longer fun for me. I couldn't generate the least little bit of enthusiasm for any of these activities. And our dinners, which had always been a time for lively conversations and kidding around, had turned into somber affairs – at least for me.

Once the children were asleep, the hours dragged by ever so slowly. I couldn't find anything that I enjoyed or that would distract me from focusing inwardly on my misery and despair. Reading was no longer an option. Books that

I previously would have found fascinating or inspiring no longer interested me, especially since depression affected my ability to concentrate on what I was reading. Television was an option, but there wasn't anything I actually enjoyed watching. I couldn't find any programs that would lift my spirits or even amuse me. In fact, when watching a comedy or listening to what was obviously a very funny joke, I couldn't even laugh. I would know intellectually that what I had heard or seen was genuinely funny, but I couldn't *feel* the humor.

My typical weekend activities also lost most of their appeal. I continued to attend swim meets and ballgames that involved my children, but they weren't the fun social events they previously had been. I didn't enjoy talking to the other parents, and I couldn't feel any of the excitement that I saw in others as we watched our children compete in the pool or on the field.

My depression also impacted my Sundays. Church had been a very important and gratifying part of my life for as long as I could remember. Growing up, my family and I were at our church every Sunday morning and most Wednesday evenings. In recent years, I had looked forward not only to worship services but also to one of the adult Sunday school classes. Led by a brilliant attorney with a lifelong interest in religion and what seemed like a photographic memory for everything he had ever read on the subject, I could count on lively, informative discussions every week. It was also in this class that I had formed some of my best friendships. But once my depression set in, I no longer looked forward to attending the Sunday school class or the worship service. I felt uncomfortable and out of place sitting among people who were obviously enthusiastic about their faith while I was mired in my dark, joyless depression, so I often opted to stay home instead.

Depression also robbed me of my ability to enjoy one of life's most basic pleasures – eating. My appetite was completely shot. Nothing appealed to me. Not even the tastiest snacks and desserts. I managed to prepare or bring home our favorite meals when my children were with me, but I couldn't enjoy what I was eating and usually failed to finish my dinner. When the children weren't with me, I didn't feel like fixing a full, healthy meal. Nor did I feel like going out to a restaurant, fearing that I might run into someone I knew who would want to talk to me. So I often skipped meals or just warmed up a can of soup. With such poor, erratic eating habits, I started losing weight, and by the time my depression hit full force, I had lost more than ten pounds.

In addition to losing interest in everything that had previously been so enjoyable – my favorite people, activities and even food – I experienced a profound sadness that was more painful and debilitating than anything I had ever experienced before.

> I experienced a profound sadness that was more painful and debilitating than anything I had ever experienced before.

This sadness was, in some respects, similar to what I had felt as I grieved the deaths of my parents just a few years earlier, but it differed in intensity and in a couple other ways. Even in the midst of grieving those losses, there were periods when

I could reminisce with my sister about the many good times we had with our parents, such as our frequent vacations to national parks where the four of us would marvel at some of God's most magnificent creations. We had warm, wonderful memories of the Great Smoky Mountains, Yellowstone, Yosemite, Grand Teton, Carlsbad Caverns and an extraordinary trip all the way to the bottom of the Grand Canyon. Despite the grief I felt, I still was able to reflect on all that they had done for me and appreciate just how blessed I was to have had them as parents, friends and mentors. I could say to myself, even as I mourned their passing, "I'm truly a very lucky person." But with my depression, there was never any reprieve from the painful sadness. It was a constant, and it kept me from thinking and feeling positively about anything from my past or anything that might lie ahead.

Also, as profoundly saddened as I was that my parents would no longer be there to provide me with their wisdom and guidance and to join me in rooting for Libby at her swim meets or Will at his baseball games or to enjoy Graham's piano recitals, their absence did not alter how I felt about myself. I still thought of myself as basically a good and fortunate person. But with the depression, I felt fundamentally changed. I was no longer confident about my value as a person, and I certainly did not feel that I could be counted among the fortunate in this world.

Another symptom of my depression, and certainly one of the worst parts of my experience, was the extreme difficulty I had sleeping. Before this, I had never had a problem with sleep. Once I had finished grading exams or reading a book or watching a television show, I could pull up the covers, close my eyes and drift off to sleep in just a few minutes. But now, I found myself lying awake in bed for what seemed like hours before finally falling asleep. One reason I was unable to fall asleep was the extremely troubling thoughts constantly rolling through my head. I couldn't stop thinking about how awful my situation was, what a terrible person I was, and how tomorrow and the next day and the following day and as far as I could see there would be only suffering and despair for me. Life seemed completely hopeless. As hard as I tried to quiet my mind, or at least shift my thoughts to other, less disturbing matters, I couldn't. The negative thoughts kept coming. Eventually, completely exhausted, I would fall asleep. But that wasn't the worst part of my sleep disturbance. The worst part was that, almost every morning, I would awaken about 4:30 and be unable to go back to sleep, even though my body was crying out for more rest. I would try every strategy I could think of, but nothing worked. My body was strangely "wired" to be awake at the same time that it was absolutely exhausted and in need of sleep. So I would lie in bed or sit in a chair staring into the darkness, waiting for the first signs of light and life. It was during these early morning hours that I felt most isolated and alone.

With so little sleep, it's not surprising that I started every day exhausted, and that by the end of the day I felt completely drained, both physically and emotionally. This was such a dramatic change for me. From childhood on, I had been blessed with a high energy level (although my parents weren't always convinced this was a blessing – at least not for them). As an adult, most mornings I would wake up refreshed and ready to teach my classes, advise students, attend committee meetings, meet with one or two patients, do a vigorous workout at the gym and still have plenty of energy to be actively involved with my children until they went to bed. After that, I typically put in another two or three hours grading exams, analyzing data or writing reports. I actually enjoyed working long hours and the sense of accomplishment that came with using my time productively. But with the depression, I never felt like I had enough energy to take on even the most basic work or family responsibilities. Tasks that I previously had performed effortlessly now seemed overwhelming. And it wasn't just a lack of energy and being easily fatigued. I felt physically weaker than I ever had before. There were times I seriously doubted that I would be able to walk the few steps from my bed to the bathroom or to the kitchen. I would swing my feet around and sit on the edge of the bed for several minutes trying to gather the strength to take those few steps, but then have to lie back down because I wasn't certain my legs were strong enough to hold me up.

And it wasn't just feeling physically weak. My emotional strength was also greatly diminished. Since high school, I had been someone to whom others would turn when they were experiencing problems or if they had serious concerns. Friends would confide in me, knowing that I would listen carefully and without passing judgment, and that I would never share what they told me with anyone else. At the university, I was often sought out by faculty and staff, as well as students, who had personal concerns. It wasn't unusual for a member of the faculty or staff to sit down with me in the cafeteria or stop me as I walked across campus to share a concern or ask for advice. But as the depression deepened and eroded my emotional strength, I found myself avoiding situations where I might run into someone who would want to talk with me about a personal matter. I didn't have the emotional strength or resilience to take on anyone else's concerns. I was too fragile emotionally. Even minor problems students were having with their courses or their friends were too much for me. I was having enough difficulty just managing my own personal issues. So I spent more and more time in my office with the door closed. There were days that I wouldn't even open my emails or listen to my voicemail messages. I simply couldn't handle the stress of someone asking me for advice or assistance.

When I was able to summon enough strength – and courage – to walk across campus to the library or cafeteria during my depressed state, I moved at a distinctly slow pace. This was quite uncharacteristic of me. As a child, I had learned to move quickly, especially when walking with my six foot, four inch father who was always in a hurry and took long, fast strides. As an adult, I continued to move rapidly most of the time, usually because I wanted to pack into each day as many activities as I could. This meant I would work on one activity (e.g., grading papers, preparing course presentations) right up to the last minute, allowing just enough time to get to my next class or appointment. But with depression sapping my energy and strength, I found myself moving very slowly most of the time. Even though I had lost weight, I felt like I was carrying an additional twenty or thirty pounds, with extra effort required to take each step. It was as if the earth's gravitational pull on me had increased. I'm not sure what I looked like to others who saw me, but I know that I felt like a frail invalid slowly shuffling down the sidewalk.

It wasn't just my body that moved slowly. My mind also was sluggish. I couldn't think with the speed and clarity that I was accustomed to. My mental abilities that had served me so well during my twenty years of formal education and more recently as a college professor were failing me. I was unable to stay focused on what I was reading. As I tried to prepare course lectures, my mind would wander off, usually returning again and again to those harsh, negative thoughts about myself, my current circumstances and the future. The same thing often happened when talking with others. I couldn't stay attentive and focused on what they were saying.

I realized just how much my mental focus and memory had deteriorated one day as I talked with a close friend who taught in the religion department. He and I were admirers of Frederick Buechner, a noted theologian and writer. In fact, this friend was the one who had introduced me to the writings of Buechner. He had been working for several years to bring the distinguished author to Stetson to give a lecture and meet with interested faculty and students. This was the year it was finally going to happen! Buechner's lecture was one of the few events I found myself looking forward to as I struggled with depression during that time. When I asked my friend to remind me exactly when Buechner would be on campus, he didn't respond immediately, but then said, with a confused, concerned look on his face, "Dan, Buechner was on campus *last* week. Didn't you know that?" Somehow, even though I had managed to come to campus each day and teach my classes – poorly, I was certain – I had completely missed what must have been several campus announcements about this distinguished guest lecturer.

Another example of how poorly my mind was functioning during this time involved a conversation I had with a staff member at the university. I was walking to my car in the parking lot one afternoon when he motioned for me to come over to the car where he was standing. When I got there, he began introducing me to his wife who was sitting in the driver's seat. As part of his introduction, he explained how helpful I had been when he had consulted with me about one of her health issues. What he was describing sounded exactly like the questions I would have asked about her health and the advice I would have given, and I definitely was the only professor on campus he would have spoken to on this particular matter. I must have been the person he consulted — but I had absolutely no memory of ever talking to him about his wife or her health. As I stood there, I realized that this earlier conversation must have occurred while I was struggling with my own health issue – depression – and having difficulty remembering events and interactions I never would have forgotten if I were not depressed.

The problems with my concentration and memory made my work as a professor even more challenging. It wasn't just that I had lost interest in teaching; I had lost confidence in myself as an intelligent, thoughtful professor.

Although, by the time of my second episode of depression, I had been promoted to the top professorial rank, published two books, and been invited to give numerous presentations on my work at professional conferences, universities and medical centers, my self-confidence was completely shattered. I felt like an absolute failure and a fraud, totally ill-equipped to engage in intelligent conversations with my fellow professors or the health professionals with whom I had been collaborating. In fact, my sense of inadequacy was so great that there were days when I truly dreaded going into the classroom, fearing that one of my students would ask the simplest, most basic question and that I would be unable to come up with the correct answer or that I would give a ridiculously incorrect response. It would then be clear to everyone in the class, and eventually word would spread throughout the university, that I was incompetent and unworthy of my position as a professor.

My sense of failure and worthlessness went well beyond my role as a college professor. One of the most painful shortcomings I felt was as a father. I loved my children immensely. They had never meant more to me than they did during this difficult time, but I knew that I had a serious problem expressing my love in a way that it could be fully felt. There was little of the warmth and enthusiasm that had been part of earlier expressions. And I felt I was failing in my responsibility to give them the care and support they needed and deserved. I was the one who should be checking in on them regularly to see how they were feeling and to offer support and to assure them that I still loved them. But too often it was the reverse. They would ask what *they* could do to help me feel better, and they were the ones who regularly told me how much they loved me. I appreciated their love and support – it helped sustain me during my darkest times – but it also reminded me of how much I was failing them. Too often I was relying on them when they should have been relying on me.

I also felt like a failure as a husband. My initial episode came shortly after my first marriage had unraveled, and with my depressive mindset, I was more than willing to absorb much of the blame. I found myself thinking over and over again about things I could have done differently.

It wasn't just feeling like a failure as a professor, father and husband that I found so disturbing. There was so much about me that seemed to have changed and I didn't like the person I had become. Where I once had thought of myself as strong and self-reliant, I now felt weak and dependent. My confidence and determination had given way to doubt and indecision. Instead of being sensitive and responsive to the needs of others, I was now focused almost exclusively on my own needs. My ability to find joy and meaning in life was gone. And then there was the terrible emotional pain. My situation seemed hopeless. I couldn't see how I could ever change back to the person I once had been, and I couldn't see a way to escape the pain.

During the darkest moments of my depression, I felt that death probably would be my only escape. And although I never seriously contemplated suicide, I did find myself thinking about death almost every day. I often thought it was likely that, like my father, I would die an early death, and there were times that didn't sound like such a terrible fate. But those thoughts only made me feel even guiltier knowing that my death would create additional hardships for my children who loved me and who had already endured far more than they deserved.

Although my training as a psychologist couldn't protect me from becoming clinically depressed, it did help me recognize the need to reach out for psychological and medical treatment. I knew that it wouldn't be wise to try to handle this by myself, so when I experienced my first depressive episode I sought the help of a psychologist I knew and trusted. I also shared my symptoms and concerns with my family physician who prescribed antidepressant medication. And, just as with the people I had treated for depression, I gradually recovered and was able to return to a full, active life. (More information about my treatment and recovery is provided in Chapter 4.)

While I knew that depression could be a chronic condition with recurring episodes, I hoped that I would be among those whose depression would not return. However, seventeen years after my initial episode, I once again found myself clinically depressed. What surprised me about this episode was that, unlike my first episode which seemed closely tied to a very stressful situation, this one seemed to come out of the blue and at a point when my life was going exceptionally well. My career was back on track, and my personal life had been on an upward trajectory ever since marrying Kim. I felt so fortunate to have enjoyed her love, companionship and support for more than a decade.

Despite the absence of any serious stressors or losses, the symptoms were just as severe as my first episode. I was back in that dark, joyless, lifeless state. I felt particularly guilty that I was not contributing much at all to the relationship with Kim. I was no longer interested in the activities we had always enjoyed doing together – weekend trips to the beach, dining out, movie nights – and I know she could feel very little warmth coming from me. I found that I couldn't enjoy, or even handle emotionally, the intimate times that had always been such a valuable part of our relationship.

As with my first episode, I knew I needed to reach out for professional help. I began seeing the psychologist who had helped me previously, and this time I sought the assistance of a psychiatrist to find the best antidepressant medication for me. I also shared what I was experiencing with my closest friends and colleagues, letting them know what I was going through and that I needed their understanding and support. Once again, I was able to recover from the depression and return to an active, productive and enjoyable life.

It has been fourteen years since my last episode of depression, and I am hopeful that I will not suffer another episode. One reason I feel hopeful is that this time, after consulting closely with my psychiatrist, I decided to stay on antidepressant medication even after I had been symptom-free for almost a year. I know this surprises some people, especially those who believe that the goal of treatment is to not be dependent on any medication or ongoing psychotherapy, but my goals are to have the energy and enthusiasm to enjoy life to the fullest and to reduce the chances of another depressive episode. If medication can help me achieve these goals, then I think staying on medication is a smart decision for me.

CHAPTER 2

A PROFESSIONAL'S PERSPECTIVE

When I began my training in psychology more than four decades ago and decided to focus primarily on depression, I had no idea that this terrible illness would strike me and my family with devastating — even deadly — consequences. As far as I knew, no one in my family had ever suffered from depression. Like most people, I had experienced periods of sadness during my adolescence and early adulthood. There had been disappointments and losses that brought sorrow into my life, but these periods of sadness never had much impact on my self-esteem, my ability to handle everyday responsibilities, or my academic and professional pursuits. The same seemed to be true of my parents. They had gone through some very difficult and discouraging times, including serious illnesses, financial struggles and the deaths of cherished family members and friends, but I had never seen either of them become seriously depressed. These difficult periods never seemed to affect their family relationships, friendships, work responsibilities or participation in church activities.

So what was it that attracted me to the study of depression and led me to devote much of my career to working with those suffering from this condition? And what are the most important lessons that I have learned from my work?

My interest in depression developed early in my training when I found myself genuinely intrigued by the tremendous impact I saw it have on the way people viewed themselves, their circumstances and their future. There was this huge discrepancy between their perceptions and what others saw. It was as if they were talking about two entirely different individuals. People who were unquestionably successful in so many ways and whose family and friends clearly loved and respected them were telling me that they were miserable failures and utterly worthless. Individuals who had so much to be grateful for and so much to live for insisted that their life was empty and the future entirely bleak.

I first began to recognize and appreciate the extent to which depression can color the beliefs and perceptions of an individual when I worked with Linda, a patient I saw during my initial year of training. Linda, a slender woman in her early thirties, appeared timid, even fearful when I met her. Her clothes hung loosely on her – the result, I learned, of recent weight loss. For most of our first few sessions, Linda sat curled up with her feet in the chair, making little eye contact and speaking so softly that I sometimes had trouble hearing what she was saying. She spent most of her time explaining how she felt like a failure in every area of her life and couldn't think of anything positive to say about herself or her situation. What she found particularly disturbing was her sense of failure in the role she valued most — being a parent. Linda described herself as an "awful mother," saying that she had neglected her son and daughter for years. She was convinced that their lives had been ruined because of her lack of attention and her troubled moods.

It wasn't difficult for me, a novice therapist, to accept what Linda was saying as largely accurate. As a single parent struggling to support herself and her children on the salary of a waitress, I knew she could have trouble finding the time and energy to be actively involved in their lives. Naïvely believing what I was being told, I allowed myself to form an impression of her children as unhappy and withdrawn, much like their mother. I might have continued to hold this impression if it were not for the time Linda brought her daughter with her to our appointment because her babysitter was ill. I must confess that I was surprised when I met this young girl.

Instead of a quiet, timid child, I found a lively, friendly little girl who was quite affectionate with her mother and who, when questioned, easily shared with me several examples of the fun things she and her mother liked to do together. And Linda seemed to come alive when she interacted with her daughter, smiling and laughing as they engaged warmly with each other. I realized that this was the first time I had seen Linda smile, and she seemed to genuinely enjoy the interaction. It didn't appear forced or unnatural. This was not at all what I had expected.

When I asked her daughter about school, I learned that she enjoyed her classes, loved her teacher and was making good grades. She also told me about all the friends she had at school. Surprised at how happy and well-adjusted she appeared to be, I realized I needed to find out more about her brother. Was he as unhappy as I had imagined, or was he, like his sister, doing well socially and academically? His sister quickly assured me that he was doing great. She said that he had plenty of friends and made good grades in all his classes. In fact, she proudly informed me that recently he had won an award as the outstanding student of the week.

My discovery of how well Linda's children were doing and how different their lives were from what she had reported prompted me to gently challenge her about her view of herself and the impact she believed she was having on others. If she was such an "awful mother," why were her children so happy and well-adjusted? Had they really suffered from neglect? Why should she feel guilty about her parenting if, in fact, her children were doing so well? Was it possible that other negative beliefs she held were inaccurate? Little by little, we chipped away at these inaccuracies and distortions. This was an important turning point in our therapy, and it was one of the most valuable lessons I learned about depression. I was beginning to understand how depression could seriously distort people's view of themselves and how, in turn, these distortions could impact their life in so many ways.

My experience with Linda also prepared me for what I encountered with one of my next patients. Andrew, a twenty-four-year-old graduate student, was accompanied to his initial visit by his wife. He had been reluctant to see a therapist, but his wife insisted that he talk to a mental health professional before he made any major decisions about his education and career. For most of our first session, Andrew sat slumped back in his chair, propping up his head with his hand and saying very little about himself or why he was there. I learned, mostly from his wife, that he was pursuing his doctorate in a prestigious, highly competitive scientific field, but was on the verge of dropping out of school, having become convinced that he lacked the intelligence to succeed in this program. He sincerely believed that there had been a mistake in the admissions process – that he never should have been admitted to the graduate program – and that soon he would be asked to leave the university because his professors would discover just how intellectually inadequate he was. He thought it would be best to withdraw from the program rather than be pushed out.

Andrew's wife, who had known him since he was a sophomore in college, was convinced that he was suffering from depression and that it was undermining his confidence and leading him to consider withdrawing from the university. She reported that he had graduated from college with high honors and been accepted into several graduate schools, all of which had offered him generous fellowships. She was certain it was not a fluke that he had been admitted to his graduate program, but she had no success convincing him of this. Andrew insisted that she did not understand the serious intellectual challenges he was facing in this program and how ill-equipped he was to succeed. It was inevitable, he believed, that he would fail. Even if his admission to the program hadn't been a mistake, he felt certain that he lacked the intelligence to succeed.

I wasn't in a position to directly challenge Andrew's beliefs about his potential to succeed in a field I knew very little about, but it was clear that he was seriously depressed and that this could be the reason for his pessimism about graduate school. After several sessions, I was able to persuade Andrew to gather some objective data rather than rely solely on his own subjective impressions. Wasn't this the approach any good scientist would take? Wouldn't it be smart to ask his academic advisor, a senior professor who had supervised numerous graduate students over the years, for a candid assessment of his academic performance thus far and his potential for future success? He was reluctant to do this, fearful of what he would hear, but he finally agreed to ask.

I felt fairly confident that Andrew would get an encouraging report, but I was still a little worried. What if Andrew's assessment of his situation was correct? How would Andrew handle bad news? Would that send him into an even deeper depression? As it turned out, I had no reason to worry. Andrew discovered that his advisor and the other faculty members considered him to be one of the best students they had ever admitted to the program, were pleased with his progress and believed that he was destined for an outstanding scholarly career. His advisor strongly encouraged him to stay in the program and, recognizing that Andrew was struggling emotionally, also urged him to continue seeing a therapist. As with Linda, this was an important turning point in our therapy, prompting us to explore other negative perceptions and beliefs that grew out of his depression. And this experience further strengthened my determination to learn more about depression.

It is important to understand that both Linda and Andrew, when describing themselves to me initially, were speaking with the deepest conviction. They genuinely believed every single negative thing they were telling me about themselves. And I heard similar distortions again and again as I worked with more depressed individuals – reports of how they were worthless, unlovable and that there was no chance life could ever improve – despite ample evidence to the contrary. I learned how these cognitive distortions were a significant aspect of depression and needed to be uncovered and addressed as part of the treatment.

Another valuable lesson I learned was that these distorted perceptions and beliefs, when combined with severe emotional pain that seems interminable, can lead to depression becoming a life-threatening condition. In fact, of all the mental disorders, depression is the most deadly, bringing with it increased risk of suicide. Each year in the United States, there are more than one million individuals who attempt suicide, and more than 45,000 of these attempts end in death. This is more than twice the number of homicides. And the suicide rate has been rising significantly. A recent analysis found that between 2001 and 2017 the suicide rate in the United States increased more than thirty percent. It now is the second leading cause of death in the 10- to 34-year-old age group and the fourth leading cause of death in those 35 to 54 years of age.

The story of Ellen, another of my former patients, illustrates how the pain of depression, coupled with the hopelessness of ever gaining relief from suffering, can lead people to view suicide as their only option. Ellen's life had not been easy. She had married early and within a few years found herself with two young children and a husband who had become increasingly abusive. Ellen had tolerated the abuse directed at her, but when he began threatening their children, she felt that she had to give up the financial security the marriage provided and move to another state. Ellen's relocation kept her and her children safe, but it also presented new challenges and hardships. It wasn't easy being a single parent, and having never completed college, she found herself trapped in a low-paying job that barely provided enough money to cover the basic expenses for her and her children. Seldom was there any extra left at the end of the month to spend on special, fun activities.

Although Ellen often felt overwhelmed as she struggled with work and family responsibilities, she managed to cope well enough emotionally until her daughter — after several heated arguments with her mother — decided to run off with her boyfriend, move to another city and cut off all contact. Ellen was devastated. She couldn't understand how her daughter could be so heartless. Feeling rejected and abandoned, Ellen fell into a serious depression and, when she began missing work, was advised by her supervisor that she needed to seek treatment.

Ellen made excellent use of her time in therapy and gradually emerged from her depression, feeling grateful that at least she still had a relationship with her son, a steady job and several good friends. I would hear from her occasionally over the next few months and she usually sounded upbeat when we talked. As you can imagine, I was quite surprised when I received a late-night telephone call from her. She apologized for waking me and promised to be brief. Ellen said that she simply wanted to say goodbye and to thank me for the care I had provided during her earlier emotional crisis. I immediately became very concerned. Why did she feel that she needed to tell me this at such a late hour? Was she okay? Did she need help? Where was she? Where was she going?

At first, Ellen did not respond to any of my questions. There was only silence on the line. Then, speaking softly, she told me that she was calling from a pay phone at a gas station. She explained that she was on her way to a nearby orange grove where she planned to park her car far enough from the highway so no one could see it, then end her life by swallowing a handful of sleeping pills and washing them down with a bottle of vodka. Ellen said that she simply could not bear the pain she was feeling any longer. Death was the only way to end her suffering. She wouldn't explain what had happened to cause her to feel life had become unbearable, but after much pleading, I was successful in persuading her to meet me at an all-night restaurant to discuss this further.

Ellen was already at the restaurant when I arrived, looking as sad and despondent as anyone I had ever seen.

It looked like she had not slept or changed clothes in several days. What I discovered as we talked was that her son had become angry with her, blamed her for the family falling apart, packed his belongings and then drove off to live with his father. At first, she thought this would be a temporary move, but it appeared that he had no plans to come home. He wouldn't even return her calls. Ellen saw these rejections by her children — the children she loved so dearly and for whom she had sacrificed so much — as permanent. She had convinced herself that she would never see either of them again, and she could not imagine how life without them could ever be worth living. How could she go on if she could not have a relationship with the only two individuals who truly mattered to her? All she could see ahead of her was a dark, painful, meaningless existence.

For the first part of our conversation that night, I simply listened as Ellen talked about how much she loved being a mother and how painful it was to be estranged from her children. Eventually, our conversation shifted to her belief that neither of her children would ever want to reconnect with her. Why was she so certain that their decisions were set in stone? Wasn't it possible that she could be wrong about this? Gradually, little by little, Ellen came around to the realization that it was impossible for her to be absolutely certain that neither of her children would ever want to have a relationship with her again. Although at this point in time she couldn't picture either of them returning to her, she had to acknowledge that someday it might happen. While this realization gave her little relief from the pain she was feeling, it did cause her to question her decision to end her life and to decide that she wanted to find a way to go on living. As long as there was the least little bit of hope that she would someday be reunited with her children, she was willing to try to carry on. But she knew she would need a lot of help and support. Would I be willing to help her? I assured her that I would be there as long as she needed.

By the end of our lengthy restaurant conversation, I felt confident that Ellen was no longer suicidal and that it would be safe to let her go back home rather than having her admitted to the hospital. She gave me the sleeping pills and bottle of vodka she had intended to use and promised to return to therapy with me later that day (by then, it was almost dawn). She also agreed to consult with a psychiatrist regarding antidepressant medication.

Ellen kept her promise to come in for her appointment and to continue therapy on a regular basis. She also followed through on my recommendation to see a psychiatrist and agreed to take the antidepressant medication he prescribed. She didn't like the idea of having to rely on medication, but she recognized that her condition was serious enough that she needed to. Over the next few months, Ellen gradually improved. An important part of her recovery was developing new relationships and goals. One important step she took was to become more active in a church she previously had attended. She also began taking college courses that could help her qualify for a promotion and boost her income.

But Ellen's story had an even happier ending than I had foreseen. First, her son discovered that life with his father wasn't what he expected and returned to live with his mother — this time with a much greater appreciation for all that she had done for him. And a few months after that, her daughter, who by then had her own daughter, decided that it was time to mend her relationship with her mother and to give her daughter and mother the opportunity to become acquainted with each other. Ellen was thrilled to be able to get to know her granddaughter, and they were able to forge an even stronger bond when Ellen's daughter took a job that required her to be out of town frequently, leaving her daughter in the care of Ellen. This was such an unexpected and amazing turn of events for Ellen! The empty, isolated life that she had felt absolutely certain was her fate – and that at one point had led her to the brink of death – had given way to renewed relationships with her children and the great joy of being a hands-on grandmother.

My experience with Ellen made a deep, lasting impression on me. I had witnessed this individual go from wanting to kill herself to thoroughly enjoying life as a mother and grandmother, and I had played a part in her recovery. I had never felt better about my work as a psychologist or more determined to help others suffering from this terrible illness.

> I had witnessed this individual go from wanting to kill herself to thoroughly enjoying life as a mother and grandmother, and I had played a part in her recovery.

Although we generally think of suicide when we talk about depression as a potentially life-threatening condition, we know that this is not the only way it can kill. Depression also can have a serious, even lethal impact on a person's physical health, aggravating and complicating other medical conditions. For example, it has been found that someone who has a heart attack and is depressed is more likely to die than the person who has a heart attack but is not depressed. It also has been found that people who are depressed have a greater risk of developing and dying from heart disease. The connection between depression and heart disease is likely due, at least in part, to the fact that depressed individuals, feeling hopeless and helpless about their situation, are less likely to take good care of themselves and to follow their doctor's treatment recommendations. My sister and I believe this is what happened to our father, and that it contributed to his death at a relatively young age.

As I mentioned earlier, at the time I began my training, I had never seen my father depressed, not even when he suffered his first heart attack at the age of forty-three. Nothing was going to slow down this six foot, four inch dynamo – not even a heart attack. Before long, he was back at work, going full speed. And with my mother's encouragement and support, he carefully followed his cardiologist's advice to improve his diet, exercise regularly and bring his weight down to a healthier level. But then, in his late fifties, following a very stressful period that culminated in the failure of one of his businesses, he became seriously depressed. This changed him dramatically. For the first time I could remember, he didn't display the confidence and determination that had characterized his life. He also lost his motivation to take good care of himself, giving up his daily walks around the neighborhood and paying little attention to his diet. It was only a few months after he became depressed that he suffered his second heart attack, this one so severe that it left him with congestive heart failure and a greatly restricted lifestyle. Just three years later, at the young age of sixty-one, he passed away. Our belief that depression contributed to our father's death was reinforced when I met with his cardiologist to discuss his medical history. His doctor, who had taken care of him for many years and knew him quite well, told me that he had been surprised at how quickly my father's heart and overall health had deteriorated following his business failure. It had been a dramatic and rapid decline, and he definitely attributed this to the stress and depression he experienced during this period.

Although I have seen again and again the devastating impact depression can have and believe it is important for everyone to understand how serious this condition can be, one of the most important lessons I have learned during my career – and a lesson that I believe needs to be shared widely – is that there is hope for those who are suffering from depression. We have effective treatments, and with proper care, most people can recover from this terrible illness. As a psychologist, it has been a great privilege to help individuals like Linda, Andrew and Ellen emerge from the dark depths of depression and recover a sense of worth, the capacity to give and receive love, the ability to feel joy again, a sense of hope, and to know that life is indeed worth living. Experiences like these have made my work and my life immensely gratifying, and they have kept me constantly searching for more opportunities to reach those affected by depression.

I was fortunate to be given just such an opportunity in 1992 when I received a grant from a charitable foundation to support the development of a health initiative focused on educating the community about depression and a number of other important health topics. Working with Drs. John Burton and Richard Bennett of Johns Hopkins, we created a program built around partnerships between medical institutions and religious congregations. A key part of this initiative was training volunteers from faith communities to serve as "lay health educators" who would coordinate educational offerings and screenings in their congregations and communities. In addition to assuming leadership for the overall program, I enjoyed conducting the training sessions on depression and then giving many of the presentations that were organized by the lay health educators. This initiative proved to be far more successful than we had expected. Congregations representing a wide range of faiths and denominations were interested in participating, and medical institutions and professionals were impressed with the large numbers of people we were able to reach. Designed to be a two-year initiative, we were so successful that we continued to receive funding year after year. By 2004, it had grown to such an extent and was consuming so much of my time that I could no longer maintain a clinical practice. While it was disappointing to have to give up my work with individual patients, it was gratifying to see how much interest there was for information on depression and other important health topics, and to know that by training volunteers we could reach thousands of people each year.

Over the twenty-seven years I have been giving these presentations on depression, I have witnessed greater and greater interest in the topic. I've been invited to speak to a number of congregations, including African Methodist Episcopal, Baptist, Catholic, Church of God, Disciples of Christ, Episcopal, Jewish, Lutheran, Methodist, Presbyterian, Seventh Day Adventist, Unitarian and United Church of Christ congregations. I've conducted workshops for hospital and police chaplains, taught Clinical Pastoral Education students, and spoken at symposia and workshops attended by clergy and lay leaders from Jewish, Christian and Muslim communities. It hasn't been unusual to have as many as seventy-five or more people attend congregational programs and for the symposia to attract more than two hundred.

I believe this growing interest reflects two trends. One is that the prevalence of depression has been increasing. When I began my clinical practice more than forty years ago, it was estimated that less than five percent of adults would experience a major depressive episode within any twelve-month period. This number has more than doubled, with a current estimated twelve-month prevalence of more than ten percent. And it is now estimated that more than twenty percent of Americans will experience at least one episode at some point during their life. That's about one in every five Americans.

Along with the increasing prevalence of depression in our communities, I have found greater openness about the topic. I am encouraged that more and more people are speaking about their experience with mood disorders, but despite this openness, there are still many people who are reluctant to talk about their depression. There are those who believe that their depression is a sign of weakness or the result of moral failure or because their faith is not strong enough. Others fear that they will not be understood and may even be criticized. Because of the stigma that many people still associate with depression and other mental illnesses, too many individuals do not receive the professional care and support that they need.

I find that my current efforts with faith communities and other organizations to erase the stigma of mental illness and to offer hope to those who are suffering from depression can be just as meaningful as my work as a psychotherapist. There are still times when I miss my clinical practice and the opportunity to work directly with patients suffering from depression, but I am constantly encouraged to continue, even expand, this work. It's tremendously gratifying to hear how the information we provide has helped people recognize their depression, overcome any sense of embarrassment about their illness, and seek professional care and the support of family and friends.

One of the first congregational programs on depression that impressed upon me the value of these programs took place following the Shabbat service at a synagogue in Florida. Working closely with her rabbi, a member of the congregation who was a graduate of our lay health educator program arranged to have a psychiatrist give a brief overview of depression. He spoke about the many important aspects of depression, describing the symptoms and some of the treatments that are available. He made a point of emphasizing that depression is a treatable condition but that people often feel so hopeless and helpless that they fail to realize how treatable it is. At the conclusion of his presentation, the rabbi came forward and encouraged the congregation to ask questions about depression and other mental disorders. After a few questions, the rabbi invited others who had questions to speak with either the psychiatrist or me after the service. Several used this opportunity not only to ask questions, but also to share their own personal struggles with depression. One of the women who spoke with me said that this was the first time she had felt comfortable talking to anyone about her depression and that she was encouraged to hear there were treatments that might help her.

Two more examples of the value of sharing information come from a recent faith-health symposium where I spoke about my personal and professional experience with depression. A young man approached me shortly after my presentation and asked if he could speak privately with me. We found a quiet corner where we could talk without being overheard or interrupted. He told me that he had attended the symposium as part of an assignment for one of his college courses, not because of a personal interest in any of the topics. But after listening to my presentation, he realized that he might be depressed. As he shared more about what he had been experiencing recently, it became clear to both of us that he was indeed depressed and that it had reached the point where he needed treatment. Fortunately, because his college provided mental health services for students, he said that he would be able to see a therapist without any concern about the cost. We agreed that was the right thing for him to do, and he promised me that he would schedule an appointment as soon as he returned to campus.

It was just a few minutes later, as I headed to the lunch line, that I was stopped by a woman who wanted to tell me that, after listening to my presentation and reviewing some of the materials she had picked up at the symposium's resource fair, she finally understood what her daughter had been going through. Furthermore, she was concerned that her daughter was not getting the treatment and support she needed. She said that she felt so strongly about this that she planned to go straight from the symposium to see her daughter, who lived several hours away, to share what she had learned and to help her find a mental health professional experienced in the treatment of depression.

An interesting and somewhat unusual opportunity to share information about depression came just a few days after the symposium when the pastor of an African American church invited me to speak to his congregation during a Sunday morning worship service. Believing that it was important for his congregation to be well-informed on depression, he insisted on letting me speak during the entire forty-five minute period he typically used for his sermon. I accepted his invitation, but I wasn't certain what to expect from the congregation. How would they feel about a psychologist delivering their Sunday morning message? As it turned out, I had no reason to worry.

The congregation was attentive throughout my presentation, and their interest in the topic was especially evident in the question-and-answer period led by their pastor that lasted another forty-five minutes. Some shared their own experiences with depression, while others asked for additional information on depression and other mental illnesses. Several times during this period, the pastor emphasized that people of faith should not be reluctant to seek professional care for depression. Spiritual care is important, he said, but so are medical and psychological care. I found this to be an especially powerful message and felt truly privileged to have been a part of this special congregational program that reached more than three hundred individuals.

One of the most moving illustrations of what can occur in a congregational setting is what I witnessed at a church where I gave a presentation immediately following the Sunday worship service. At the conclusion of my presentation, there was an opportunity for questions and comments. One person had a question about some of the medications for depression. Another asked for advice about talking with a family member who appeared to be depressed. Then, a woman asked if she could take a few minutes to share her personal experience with depression. Everyone listened attentively as she described how painful and difficult her life had been for much of the past year. She talked about her feelings of worthlessness and hopelessness, and how uncomfortable it was to be around others because she was certain they could never understand what she was experiencing. These were some of the feelings that had kept her away from the church and people she loved. But she had decided to come back to church that day, hoping that she might gain a better understanding of what she was going through and learn where to turn for help. Having listened carefully, she now felt, for the first time in months, that there was hope for her. She felt that coming back to church and learning more about depression had been an important first step on what would be a healing journey. She also wanted to express her gratitude to her church for sponsoring the program and for creating a safe, welcoming space where she could feel comfortable speaking openly about her illness. This was gratifying to hear, but it was what happened next that I found so beautiful and inspiring. As the program ended, several members of the congregation gathered around this woman, warmly embracing her physically and with loving words. They let her know how much they cared about her and how they wanted to support her on her healing journey, offering to be with her every step of the way.

When I reflect on these and other similar experiences, I am reminded of the words of theologian Frederick Buechner, who has said, "The place God calls you to is the place where your deep gladness and the world's deep hunger meet." (*Wishful Thinking: A Theological ABC*) I see again and again that there is great hunger for information on depression, and nothing brings me greater joy than to know that I have been able to provide information that will help someone find the care and support they need to recover from this terrible illness.

CHAPTER 3

A FATHER'S PERSPECTIVE

I can't remember any year I looked forward to with greater anticipation and excitement than 1976. If everything went as planned, I would successfully defend my doctoral dissertation, complete my clinical internship, receive my Ph.D., and embark on a career as a clinical psychologist. As excited as I was about these potential accomplishments (and they all did come to pass right on schedule), I was even more excited about another expected event – the birth of our first child, Libby. The big day finally arrived on February 21. I can't express how amazing it felt to be at her birth, then hold her in my arms. It only took minutes to feel a tremendously strong bond with this beautiful child and to begin imagining all the great times we would have together. I felt so proud to be her father and so hopeful about her future. But there also was the anxiety that goes along with being a new parent. I was going to be responsible for the health and safety of this child. Would I be able to protect her from diseases, injuries and people who might do her harm? Would I be wise enough and strong enough to guide her and support her as she moved from childhood to adolescence and then into adulthood?

Although Libby's mother, Mary, and I made our fair share of mistakes, I believe that we can rightfully say we did a good job protecting and supporting Libby for most of her childhood — or for at least the first ten years. We took all the proper precautions to make our home safe, made sure she was always strapped securely into her car seat, and took her to the pediatrician for well and sick visits. When we both had to be away from home, we made certain that she was left in the care of devoted family members or babysitters that we had thoroughly vetted. When we moved to Florida – where there are lakes and pools aplenty – we made sure to sign Libby up for swim lessons as soon as possible. She was only a year old when we discovered she was a natural swimmer – and a powerful one at that.

When it was time for Libby to begin preschool, our protective instincts kicked in even more. We wanted to make sure we found the school that would be best for her education and overall development. After carefully checking into a number of schools, we decided that the best option was a preschool where one of our friends was the director. Libby enjoyed her time at the school and received an excellent education, but the following year we had to search for another school when our family moved to DeLand, Florida where I had accepted a faculty position at Stetson University.

The move to DeLand seemed to be good for the family. It had the feel of a small town where everyone knows everyone else. There were regular fun activities for families – festivals and picnics in the park, Easter egg hunts, fireworks on the Fourth of July, an annual Christmas parade through the middle of town – and when hurricanes or other crises struck, the community seemed to come together as one. We also found Stetson to be a close-knit community that offered a number of events and programs that the children of faculty and staff enjoyed. The move also brought us closer to my parents who had moved to DeLand a few years before, and we were still close enough to Orlando that our children would be able to visit their maternal grandparents and cousins regularly. It seemed like an ideal setting to raise our children.

As I talked with my new colleagues about the schools in DeLand, I learned that many considered the best option to be the preschool at First Presbyterian Church. This sounded ideal since we were Presbyterians and planned to become members of that church. It also had the benefit of being just a few blocks from my campus office, which made it easy for me to attend any special programs or just to observe her interacting with her teachers and classmates.

We couldn't have been more pleased with our decision to enroll Libby at First Presbyterian's preschool and kindergarten. It was there that she established lasting friendships with several of her classmates. And it also was where she formed a special bond with one of her teachers who remained a close friend and one of her strongest advocates. When it came time for Libby to enter first grade, we once again had to make a decision about what would be best for her. One of our concerns was that Libby was quieter and more reserved than many children. We wanted to make sure that she was in a school where she would get the attention and support we felt she needed. As we had done before, we looked carefully at the options before deciding that she could receive an excellent education and the individual attention she needed in the public elementary school near our home.

Libby's elementary school years were mostly happy times. She did well in her classes, and she had good friends at school and church. Additionally, by the time she turned seven, she also had two siblings – her sister Graham, born in 1978, and her brother Will, born in 1982. Libby loved being a big sister, and she was always protective of her siblings (although they have many stories about the times she teased or tricked them). One of her favorite activities was to play teacher for Graham and Will. On weekends, I would take them to campus and let them use one of the empty classrooms next to my office. There, Libby would give spelling lists or arithmetic problems to her siblings, help them with their assignments and then grade their work.

I was fortunate that my teaching schedule at the university gave me the flexibility to be involved in the lives of my children to a greater extent than most working parents. As long as I was willing to do much of my course preparation and grading in the evenings after the children were in bed, I could get away from campus in time to pick them up from school and attend many of their afternoon activities. My academic schedule also gave us plenty of time together during the summer months, including memorable vacations in the mountains of North Carolina, visits to interesting historical sites in New England and frequent trips to the beach.

One of the most significant developments during this period was Libby joining the swim team at the local YMCA when she was seven. Immediately, it became apparent that she was a remarkably gifted swimmer. It was such an amazing experience to watch our young daughter confidently step up onto the starting block, spring forward at the sound of the starter's gun, and then move swiftly through the water with smooth, strong strokes and powerful kicks, almost always finishing ahead of the other swimmers. It wasn't long before she was winning numerous medals and trophies for her swimming. By the time she was ten, she was nationally ranked in eight events in her age group, including being number one in the country in both the 50- and 100-yard freestyle. In 1987, she was honored as the Florida Swimmer of the Year for her age group.

Although Libby was blessed with natural athleticism, it is important to understand — especially in light of her later struggles with depression — that she could not have succeeded at the level she did if it were not for her strong desire to win and her commitment to the time, effort and energy it took to compete with the very best. That meant several hours of practice after school every day and morning practices during the summer months. Some days, as she prepared for major competitions, she would swim as much as four miles. We could support her by making sure she got to her practices and swim meets, but it was up to her to put in the hard work if she wanted to be the best. There is no question that at this point in her life Libby had a strong competitive spirit. She was dedicated, disciplined and determined to succeed.

Unfortunately, at the same time Libby was receiving numerous honors for her swimming, she was becoming more and more aware that all was not well at home. Mary and I were not able to shield her and her siblings from the relationship problems we were having. Libby could feel the tension and, like many first-born children, tried to play peacemaker and assure Graham and Will that everything would be okay. Despite counseling, our efforts to keep our marriage together eventually failed. This meant that Libby, Graham and Will would not be able to experience the degree of stability and security that their mother and I had when we were growing up. Both of us were fortunate to have been raised in families where the marriages were strong and where we were able to spend plenty of time with both of our parents almost every single day.

There was no way to escape the painful realization that the divorce was going to be hard on our children. It was clear that they loved both of us and wanted both of us to be involved in their lives on a regular and frequent basis. Libby was particularly vocal about wanting to make sure that our custody arrangement would allow her to spend plenty of time with me. The bond I felt the day she was born had strengthened greatly over the years. One of the reasons that we had become close was that she and I were similar in temperament. Both of us were introverts who preferred quiet, one-on-one or small group interactions. If we found ourselves in a large, noisy gathering, we often would go off together to explore the neighborhood, toss a Frisbee or just talk with each other.

Another reason we had grown closer over the years was our shared interest in sports and physical activities, especially swimming. At the pool or the beach, Libby and I were usually the first ones in the water. As much as I treasured this close relationship with Libby, I would learn much later that it had a downside, too. Because Libby never wanted to disappoint me, she often kept me in the dark when she was having some of her most serious problems.

Mary and I – trying to make the best of a difficult situation – committed to staying in DeLand as long as our children were in school. We also developed a shared custody arrangement that allowed the children to spend several days every week with each of us. Fortunately, we lived only a few miles apart, but that didn't mean it was easy on the children. They had to pack up personal items and school materials each time they moved to the other parent's home. They also found there were different rules at each home. And then, just a few months after our divorce was finalized, Libby, Graham and Will faced an additional challenge when their mother remarried, bringing a stepfather and three stepbrothers into their lives. Complicating this further for Libby was the fact that her new stepfather had been, and would continue to be for several years, her swim coach. Libby would later tell me that she often felt guilty because it was her swimming that first brought her mother and her stepfather together. As much as I assured her that she was in no way responsible for the breakup of our marriage, she had a hard time letting go of the guilt she felt.

There was another adjustment that Libby had to make around this time, and it was one that worried her mother and me as we remained concerned about guiding and supporting her. She would be entering middle school. This meant that she would be interacting with a much larger group of students than she had experienced in elementary school where we knew most of her friends and their parents. We would be less informed about what was going on in her life, and we could not expect to have the same degree of influence over her decisions and activities. It's a loss of influence that I imagine most parents feel as their children mature, but that doesn't make it any easier to accept, especially when you have been responsible for creating some of the turmoil and stress your children are experiencing during this critical period. Our commitment to protecting Libby remained strong, but our ability to do so was growing weaker.

While I was concerned about losing much of the influence over Libby's life, I found it important to remind myself that because of the divorce, the shuttling back and forth between two homes, and the introduction of new family members, she also was losing some of the control over her life. This could not have been easy, especially for a child who liked her life to be quiet and orderly.

One change we noticed during Libby's middle school years was that she became more critical of herself, especially her appearance. Graham recalls that she had been known as one of the "pretty" girls during her elementary school years and continued to be viewed that way by her middle school peers, but that's not how she saw herself. She began talking about being fat, even though at no point in her life was she ever overweight. But otherwise, Libby appeared to be doing well. She had a number of close friends, handled her school work without any problems, continued to excel athletically, and seemed to enjoy the time she and her siblings spent with me. After their homework was done, we often went on "mystery rides" in the evening, exploring the various neighborhoods and backroads of our community. I'm sure that one reason they enjoyed these rides was because we never failed to end up at their favorite ice cream store. The four of us also enjoyed several vacations together during this time, visiting cousins in Atlanta and friends from graduate school in New England, touring Washington, D.C. and Williamsburg, and spending at least a week at the beach each summer. I remember Libby always having a great time during these trips, and also continuing to be very protective of Graham and Will.

This was the period when I discovered that Libby was also looking out for me much of the time. She seemed genuinely concerned about me and eager to be of help as I faced the various challenges of being a single parent. One of the best examples was when I was "asked" (i.e., strongly encouraged) by Stetson University's president and provost to become dean of students. Although this would mean a significant increase in salary, I would have to give up teaching the courses I enjoyed so much and reduce the number of patients I was seeing in my clinical practice. Most importantly, my administrative responsibilities would cut into the time I would have with my children. Although I didn't want to take on this new role, I was feeling pressured. The university had experienced serious problems in the student affairs department and needed new leadership, and I felt confident that I could handle the challenges.

I can remember very clearly discussing this with my children as we enjoyed an after school snack of french fries and soft drinks at a local restaurant. After listening carefully, Libby asked me two simple questions that cut right to the heart of the matter: Did I really *want* to take this position? And, didn't I enjoy spending time with her and Graham and Will? After answering "no" to the first question and "yes" to the second, she asked very simply and directly, "Then why would you take the job?" It was then that I realized Libby was seeing this important issue far more clearly and thoughtfully than some of my friends and colleagues I had consulted. This would not have been the right move for me. Even if I had succeeded in my role as dean, I would have been resentful about what I had given up. I was so grateful that she had spoken up, and I appreciated her ability to see what would be best for me. What I would soon realize was that while Libby was very protective of others, including me, she was not nearly as good about protecting herself. And while she could help me make good decisions, she was about to enter a very difficult time in high school when she would make some highly questionable, and at times costly, decisions for herself.

It wasn't too long after Libby started high school that we began to see signs of depression. One of the first signs was that she began struggling with school. While it's certainly not unusual for teenagers to have difficulty adjusting to their high school courses, Libby's struggles were different from those of her classmates. Her difficulties and unhappiness went well beyond the classroom. There was a pervasive sadness and almost complete apathy. She no longer enjoyed any part of her school experience or even her time away from school. She passed up opportunities to go out with friends or family on weekends, instead withdrawing into her room. It was virtually impossible to find anything that interested her or that would elicit a smile or laugh. Even food had lost much of its appeal, resulting in a noticeable loss of weight. And there were frequent complaints about being tired, even though she was sleeping far more than usual.

Also noticeable was how Libby's outlook on the future and life in general became overwhelmingly negative. It was unusual to hear her say anything positive about anyone, even her longtime friends. Instead, she seemed to have something critical to say about everyone. What I found particularly worrisome was that she was aiming more and more criticism at herself, often talking about how she was unattractive and stupid. When given compliments or reminded of her successes, she dismissed them as meaningless. And she no longer spoke in hopeful terms about the future. There were no more conversations about college, careers or relationships. In fact, she didn't appear to have any future plans or anything to look forward to. At times, she even hinted that she wasn't sure her life was worth living.

This also was the period when Libby began to experiment with drugs. Friends who knew her during that time believe that she turned to drugs primarily in response to her depression as a way of self-medicating. They could see that she was hurting emotionally and wanted to take something that would alter how she felt.

> Mary and I recognized that this wasn't just teenage moodiness. It was far more serious.

Mary and I recognized that this wasn't just teenage moodiness. It was far more serious. This was a clinical depression that was impacting every area of her life, and she seemed to be sinking deeper and deeper. As parents, this was frightening to watch. We could offer her our love and support, but we knew this was not enough. We feared that, without treatment, her condition could get much worse and possibly even become life-threatening. Although Libby didn't want to admit that she needed to see a psychologist or psychiatrist, we insisted and were grateful that we did. The results weren't immediate, and at one point she even needed to be hospitalized for a few days. But Libby gradually recovered from her depression, and she was able to once again enjoy activities with family and friends, and handle her coursework without much difficulty. It was such a relief to see her smiling and laughing and enjoying being with others. The "old" Libby was back!

There was another significant development in Libby's life during her high school years. This was when I began dating Kim. Knowing how difficult it had been for Libby to deal with the addition of a stepfather and three stepbrothers to her family, Kim and I tried to keep our time together mostly separate from my time with the children.

Kim didn't want them to feel like they would have to compete with her for my time and attention. After we had been dating for a little over two years, we began to seriously think about getting married. We weren't in a rush to marry, but we were eager to spend more time together and felt that we were ready to make a life-long commitment to each other.

Before we made any wedding plans, I shared my thoughts about marrying Kim with my children. I was particularly concerned with how Libby would feel about adding one more member to the family. The three of them responded positively, but to be honest, I don't think that Libby was thrilled with the idea. Still, she insisted that I deserved to be happy, and she knew how much I enjoyed being with Kim. I would later learn that, prior to the wedding, Libby had issued a "warning" to Kim. They were in the car together, and the topic of our marriage came up. Libby informed Kim that she was fine with the marriage, but that Kim "better not ever hurt my father." Once again, Libby was protecting those she loved.

Libby's junior year of high school brought a new, serious challenge – she found out she was pregnant. Her response to this was one of purpose and determination. She informed us that she definitely wanted the child and that she would not allow becoming a mother to interfere with her education. Libby also chose to marry her baby's father at this time. Although I was worried about the impact these life-changing events would have on her, I was impressed by the determination and dedication that Libby showed. Her daughter, Jordan, was born a little before Christmas in 1993 and immediately brought great joy into Libby's life and into the lives of many others. Libby clearly relished being a mother, and with the help of family and friends, she was able to graduate from high school on schedule and then enroll in college.

Handling a full course load at Stetson University while having the responsibility of a young child presented many challenges for Libby, but she never asked for special treatment. Upon discovering that she had a young child, several of her professors told me that they wished she had shared this information with them. They had no idea that her occasional absences were usually due to having a sick child. But Libby didn't want to make excuses or be treated differently. The drive, discipline and determination she had shown during her childhood years were evident once again.

Libby graduated from Stetson with a degree in teacher education, an obvious career choice for someone whose parents were both educators. It also would be relatively easy for her to find a job, something she would need to help provide for her young family. She was able to obtain a position as a teacher at a private school; however, she soon discovered that it was not as rewarding as she had hoped. Teaching twenty spirited young children was not the ideal work situation for someone who was introverted and preferred one-on-one or small group interactions. Along with the job-related stress, there were difficulties at home that multiplied over time. Eventually, Libby and her husband separated, then tried to get back together a couple times, but finally concluded that their marriage could not be saved.

Libby seemed to rebound after her divorce. She stayed in closer contact with family members, particularly her sister, Graham, who had recently transferred to Stetson.

Libby and Jordan lived with Graham during this post-divorce period, which I think was one of her happier times.

Eventually, Libby began dating and seemed to enjoy going out occasionally. One of my clearest and favorite memories is the time Kim and I met Jordan, Libby and her date at the county fair. One of the reasons this memory stands out is because Libby was having such a great time. She enjoyed going on rides with Jordan, eating cotton candy and popcorn, and kidding around with her date. It had been a long time since I had seen Libby having this much fun. I hoped this was a sign that her depression was well behind her and would never return, even though I knew we couldn't count on that.

A few years after her divorce, Libby started dating Mike, a former high school classmate. This relationship appeared to be good for her. Mike was intelligent and industrious, had a steady job, and did not seem discouraged that Libby had a young daughter. In addition to love and companionship, this relationship also offered a degree of stability and security that she had not enjoyed for years. You can imagine how happy we were when Libby and Mike decided to get married.

Within a year of their marriage, Collin was born. Libby and Mike were both thrilled to have a son, and Jordan enjoyed being a big sister, helping with his care just like Libby had helped care for Graham and Will. It looked like Libby's life was moving in a good direction. She had a stable family with two beautiful children, and she finally found a job she enjoyed – working as a receptionist in a physician's office. It was quiet and orderly, and everyone who worked there seemed to like Libby and be pleased with her performance. I was delighted when one of my university colleagues, who had met Libby when he went for his medical appointment, commented on how cheerful and helpful she had been. This was more confirmation, I thought, that Libby was doing well.

But all was not well with Libby – she was abusing prescription drugs. The problem was serious enough that she lost her job and entered a residential treatment program. Although initially resistant to treatment, Libby successfully completed the program, and we were hopeful that she could get back on track with her life. We knew that she would face some challenges, but all of us were ready to support her when she did.

The following years seemed to generally go well for Libby, Mike and the children. We saw them often — getting together for dinner on the weekend, trips to the zoo, vacations at the beach and holiday gatherings. Libby appeared to be in good spirits during the times we spent with her. When I would stop by her home after work to visit, I usually found her gardening, helping Jordan with her schoolwork, playing games with Collin or engaged in her latest arts and crafts project. I was encouraged by what I saw and by our upbeat conversations. Any complaints or frustrations she discussed seemed typical for a young working mother. I remained concerned about the possibility that her depression would return, but I didn't see any evidence that it had.

Mike also saw this as mostly a happy time for Libby and the entire family. They particularly enjoyed doing things with Graham and her family – backyard cookouts, boating on the river, trips to Orlando to visit grandparents and cousins, and holiday gatherings. But looking back, Mike believes there may have been signs that Libby was beginning to struggle with depression again. He remembers periods when she complained about being exhausted, despite spending more and more time in bed, and there were times she didn't have the energy to engage in many of the activities she previously had enjoyed with Jordan and Collin. He would try to talk with her about how she was feeling, but she wouldn't say much and didn't want anyone's help.

One of the happiest developments during this time was the discovery that Libby was pregnant with a little girl. Unfortunately, this pregnancy did not go as smoothly as her two previous pregnancies, and Kamryn was born three months prematurely. Luckily, everything turned out well, and after three months in the neonatal intensive care unit, Kamryn came home from the hospital a healthy, happy baby.

Libby was excited to have Kamryn home with the rest of the family, but over the next year she began developing some of the same symptoms of depression she had experienced as a teenager – a persistent sadness, less and less interest in activities she previously enjoyed, loss of appetite, sleep difficulties, exhaustion, extreme self-criticism, pervasive pessimism – and this time the symptoms were more severe and debilitating. Additionally, she was increasingly irritable and short-tempered, often saying things that she later regretted. It became clear that Libby was not going to be able to pull out of the depression by herself, and several of us encouraged her to seek professional care. What happened next is unclear. If she did see a psychologist or psychiatrist, she didn't tell anyone. But we do know that many of her symptoms persisted and seem to have contributed to marital problems that reached the point where Libby and Mike decided it would be best for them to live apart.

Libby then went through a very difficult period as she tried to establish a new home for herself and the children. She always had good intentions as she worked toward this goal, but some of her decisions proved to be quite unwise and created even more difficulties. Finding the right living arrangement was particularly challenging. She ended up changing her residence several times over the course of a year, and often had to call on me and other family members to help her move or to cover some of her bills. One benefit of her needing my assistance was that I had more opportunities to talk with her and to impress upon her the need for treatment of her depression. When she said that she was reluctant to see a mental health professional because of the expense and transportation problems, I assured her that I would gladly cover the cost of her visits and any medication, and that I could even take her to her appointments. I was greatly relieved when she finally accepted my offer and arranged to see a psychiatrist in Orlando. Although it was an hour-long drive each way, I didn't mind since it gave us a chance to talk more about her current situation and to work on future plans.

Gradually, Libby's life began to smooth out, probably due at least in part to the fact that she was taking her antidepressant medication regularly. One of the most positive developments during this time was that she was able to find a good living situation for herself and the children, sharing a house with a friend she had known in high school. He was also a single parent with three young children, and the house was large enough that Libby and her children could have their own rooms. One of the advantages of this house was that it came with a large yard, allowing Libby to pursue her love of gardening. It was reassuring to see her once again enjoying one of her favorite hobbies. Often when I stopped by to visit, she would be planting or watering flowers, or adding some personal decorative touches to the house. She seemed calm and relaxed when we talked – much more so than she had been for a long time – and she appeared to be genuinely happy with her situation. Each time I saw her, I came away encouraged about her mental health and overall well-being.

Just as I was starting to feel comfortable with Libby's situation, I faced a major career decision. I had been a professor at Stetson University for more than three decades and loved working with the students, but Dr. Richard Bennett, my longtime collaborator on my medical-religious partnership work, had become president of Johns Hopkins Bayview Medical Center and invited me to join him. He was eager to bring our community health model to Baltimore and offered me the position of special advisor to the president. This was an amazing opportunity. I would be a member of the executive team at a hospital that was part of an internationally renowned health system, and I also would have academic appointments at the Johns Hopkins University School of Medicine.

I remember quite clearly the Saturday I drove to Libby's house to discuss this opportunity with her. She was outside, watering the flowers that lined the driveway. We stayed outside as we talked. I told her about the job offer, uncertain how she would respond. I didn't have to say much before she spoke up and said, "Dad, you definitely should take the offer. I know you've passed up other opportunities because of me and Graham and Will, and you shouldn't pass on this one. I'll miss you, but I'll be okay. I promise."

I accepted Dr. Bennett's offer, and Kim and I began planning our move to Baltimore. Libby and I promised that we would stay in touch with regular phone calls, and I assured her that we would return to Florida for the Christmas holidays so that we could spend time together with the rest of our family.

My initial long-distance phone conversations with Libby were largely reassuring. It sounded like she and her children were still doing well, but then I had trouble reaching her for a couple weeks. I left several messages, but she didn't return my calls. I finally heard from her, and she said she was fine, but then told me that she had moved out of the house where she had been living and was now staying with a family down the street. This worried me. Why would she move out of the home that had seemed so good for her and the children? I soon learned that she had a new boyfriend and had moved in with him. I didn't find this comforting, especially when it became increasingly difficult to reach her by phone. I'm not sure what I could have done if I had been in Florida, but I felt especially helpless being more than 800 miles away.

Meeting Libby's new boyfriend over the Christmas holidays did little to calm my worries, but she insisted she was happy. I was able to have a few private moments with her and tried to get her to tell me more about this new relationship, but all she would say was that she was doing fine and that I didn't need to worry. I wasn't convinced, but I didn't know what else I could say or do. This is one of the most frustrating and worrisome aspects of being a parent of an adult child who could be having serious problems. There's little you can do other than offer your support and then pray they will be okay.

Still, there was plenty of good news as the family gathered. Jordan, Collin and Kamryn were healthy and happy, and Jordan was on track to graduate from high school in June. Graham and her husband, Eric, were expecting their third child, and Will and his longtime girlfriend, Katherine, were discussing wedding plans. It felt great to have everyone together, and all of us promised to return to Florida in June to help celebrate Jordan's graduation.

It was difficult to stay in touch with Libby during the time between our Christmas vacation and Jordan's graduation in June. She and her boyfriend moved several times, and she hadn't been able to find a steady job. I also was hearing reports from family and friends in Florida that Libby was often depressed. But every time we talked, Libby insisted she was fine, and she sounded like she was doing well. She never complained about her circumstances or mentioned that she was unhappy. In fact, she always wanted to talk more about how Kim and I were doing. Did we like Baltimore? How was my work going?

Jordan's graduation was a joyous occasion for the entire family. We were so proud as we watched her walk across the stage and receive her diploma. On the wall of my office, I have a photo from that day — Jordan in her green graduation gown standing next to her smiling mother who has Kamryn in her arms and Collin standing right beside her. It was a beautiful, uplifting sight. Later that day, we gathered at Mary's home to continue the celebration. Little did I know that this would be the last happy occasion I would spend with all three of my children.

> Little did I know that this would be the last happy occasion I would spend with all three of my children.

The next few months were worrisome. Although Libby always insisted when we talked that she was okay, I was getting reports that her behavior was often irrational and erratic. I would find out later that there had been many disturbing developments during that period, including Mike becoming so concerned about the safety of their children that he felt he had to petition the court to gain temporary custody.

In the meantime, I was wrapping up my first year at Johns Hopkins. We successfully launched several community health programs, and I was finding my work even more rewarding than I had hoped. Before I started working on programs for my second year, Kim and I were able to get away and enjoy the beauty of Shenandoah National Park, one of the many parks I had visited with my parents and sister. We then returned to Baltimore, ready for another busy year. Within hours of our return, I received a call from Mary. Will had spent the weekend at her home, and she and Libby had driven him to the airport in Orlando so that he could return to Nashville. On their way back to DeLand, while going seventy miles per hour on the interstate, Libby had taken off her seatbelt, opened the car door and tried to jump out. The only reason she failed was because her mother grabbed her hair and pulled her back in. As you can imagine, Mary was terrified and confused. Libby couldn't explain why she had done this. All she could say was, "Everything went black."

We both agreed that this called for an emergency psychiatric evaluation. Libby protested, but we insisted. She was admitted to an inpatient facility for observation and evaluation. A few days later, the staff determined she was no longer actively suicidal and released her.

I wish I had found the results of this evaluation reassuring, but I didn't. I remained very concerned. The only encouraging news was that Libby would be able to stay with her mother until she found a better housing situation and could get into a treatment program.

It was only a few days later that I received another call from Mary. This time the news was even worse. Libby, while home alone, had tried to kill herself by drinking muriatic acid she found in the cabinet where the pool supplies were kept. She had been taken to the local hospital, but the damage to her esophagus and lungs was so severe that she was transferred to Shands Hospital at the University of Florida in Gainesville. It wasn't clear if she would survive.

Kim and I immediately flew to Charlotte where we met Graham and Will, and then drove straight to the hospital where we joined Jordan and Mary. We were told that the doctors were uncertain about Libby's odds of surviving or – if she were to survive – what her life would be like. Each of us was allowed to spend a little time with Libby as she laid in her hospital bed, unresponsive and with tubes and wires connecting her to machines that were keeping her alive. I would like to think that she heard at least some of what I was telling her about our love and hopes for her, but there was no way for me to know if she did.

At the same time that we were doing everything we could to make sure Libby was getting the medical care she needed, we were also finalizing arrangements to be in Nashville for Will's wedding where I would be serving as his best man – one of the greatest honors of my life. Graham and Jordan were also to be part of the wedding party. I had never experienced the range of extreme emotions I was feeling. Here I was, so proud of my son and wanting to do everything I could to make his wedding the happy, festive occasion it should be, while feeling tremendous heartache knowing that my daughter was lying in an intensive care unit tethered to a ventilator. Nothing can prepare you for a situation like that. Thankfully, I was able to carry out my responsibilities as best man and enjoy the wedding and reception. But the moment I stepped away from the reception, I broke down. All I could think about was Libby in her hospital room almost 600 miles away.

After almost a month at Shands Hospital, Libby's doctors felt she was medically stable enough to be transferred back to the hospital in DeLand where family and friends could visit more often. We were encouraged by this development, but the doctors were still uncertain about her chances of recovery. All we could do was pray and hope for the best, uncertain exactly what that would look like. The doctors tried to wean her off the ventilator several times, but never succeeded. When we discussed with doctors and case managers what the options would be, they felt the best Libby could hope for would be to stay in a skilled nursing facility – perhaps for the rest of her life. They were not optimistic about her ever living independently again. I can't even express how heartbreaking this was. Here was this beautiful young woman, who in her prime swimming years competed with and often defeated other swimmers who went on to win gold medals in the Olympics, but now could not even get out of her hospital bed by herself. She would never get into a swimming pool again, not even to just splash around with her children.

Still, through all this sorrow, there were occasional bright moments. Whenever I visited Libby, she would greet me with a big smile and then mouth the words, "How are you?" and "I love you." She always wanted to hear about my work and life. Jordan said the same was true when she visited her mother. Somehow, despite being confined to a hospital bed and dependent on a ventilator to keep her alive, she was still able to radiate warmth and love. It was one of the greatest gifts I could have received.

Early on January 14, 2013, I received a text from Mary. The hospital had called – Libby's situation was dire and I should get there as soon as possible. But before I could even get out of the apartment and to the airport, there was another call – Libby had died.

I flew down to Florida to meet with Mary, Jordan, Graham and Will to make funeral arrangements. It was during these discussions that Graham and Will encouraged me to speak openly at the memorial service about Libby's struggles with depression. They wanted some good to come out of this tragic loss. As I recounted in my introductory chapter, I spoke candidly, and the response was overwhelmingly positive. People agreed that it was important to bring the subject of depression out of the darkness and into the light.

The day after Libby's memorial service, we took her ashes to a cemetery in Orlando where they could be placed near her grandfather's grave. As the family gathered around, we watched Collin, only nine years old, gently place the box with his mother's ashes into the ground, lovingly lay a rose on top and then slowly scoop dirt over the box. It is a scene that will remain with me forever, and it is one of the memories that drives me to continue my work raising awareness about depression. No child should have to experience what Jordan, Collin and Kamryn have been through. Mike has continued to be a great father to the three of them, and grandparents, aunts and uncles, cousins, and close friends have stepped in to offer love and support. But it still doesn't take away the fact that they have been deprived of many years of the love and concern and touch of their mother.

Libby's death left our family with a number of unanswered questions. We knew that her depression was the major factor contributing to her suicide, but we weren't certain what other factors played a role. And Jordan, who had two children in the years following her mother's death, had trouble understanding how a mother could take her own life, knowing that she would be leaving behind her children.

To try to find answers to some of our questions, I traveled to Florida six years after Libby's death to meet with her mother, Mike and Jordan to discuss what Libby's life had been like in the months leading up to her suicide attempts. We got together on what would have been Libby's forty-third birthday. I also talked with Graham and Will, exploring some of the same questions and concerns. Although we didn't get answers to all our questions, I felt we gained a better understanding of Libby's last few months and learned some important lessons.

First, although some might be tempted to interpret Libby's suicide as evidence that she did not love her children very much, we know that this is not true. There is no question in my mind – or the minds of other family members – about Libby's love for her children. From the moment Libby learned that she was pregnant with Jordan, nothing was more important in her life than being a good mother. And when she was not depressed, she was a great mother. She loved being actively engaged with her children – swimming with them, taking them to the zoo or playground, helping them with their school work, and then gently tucking them into bed each night and softly telling them how much she loved them. She cherished these times with each of her children. It was because of Libby's deep love for her children that her sense of failure as a mother was especially painful. She hadn't been able to provide them with the stable, secure home life that she had wanted for them. She hadn't been able to provide for them financially like she had wanted to.

But it wasn't just her inability to provide for her children that made her feel like a failure. It was also her belief that during her depressed periods she had seriously neglected them. She felt that she had been inattentive and unresponsive to their needs, and that there were times when she had said or done very hurtful things. She knew that there had been occasions when she embarrassed her children in front of their friends.

Failing as a teacher or receptionist or even as a wife could be disappointing and hurtful for Libby, but none of these could compare to her sense of failure as a mother. Nothing was more precious to her than her children, and no memories were happier than those of her with the children during the good times.

The more Libby struggled with depression, the guiltier she felt about the harm she believed she had caused her children and the more pessimistic she became about ever being a good mother to them. She felt that she didn't have the energy to take proper care of them, and she couldn't escape the realization that some of her words and actions had been hurtful, although I'm certain that she greatly exaggerated the negative impact they had. She even questioned her judgment as a mother, and her depression often distorted what she saw and heard. The best example of this, and one I still find painful to think about, is the time Mike, out of genuine concern for the safety of their children, had to petition the court to grant him temporary custody. Libby viewed this as permanent. In her mind, Collin and Kamryn had been taken away from her *forever*. It was only in these conversations six years after her death that I learned the week before her suicide attempt she had told someone, "I might as well kill myself – I've lost my kids."

I also was reminded in my discussions with Mary, Mike, Jordan, Graham and Will how much Libby tried to hide her problems and concerns from us – particularly from me. Jordan described how there were times when her mother had not showered or changed out of her clothes or moved off the couch for an entire day, but would quickly shower, brush her hair, and put on clean clothes and her makeup when she heard that I would be stopping by. She always wanted me to think that she was doing well and to be proud of her.

It also appears that stigma often interfered with Libby obtaining the treatment she needed for her depression. Even though Mary and I viewed depression as a medical illness, as did Graham and Will, she was never able to view it this way. In her mind, depression was entirely different from other illnesses, such as the asthma she had since childhood. Like most children and adults, Libby talked openly about her asthma and didn't feel embarrassed or ashamed to use her inhaler when needed. But like so many others, she viewed depression differently. She didn't want to be seen as having a mental illness, particularly one that required medication or seeing a therapist on a regular basis. She wanted to be viewed as "normal."

I think the most important lesson I learned from reflecting on the months leading up to Libby's suicide attempts is that our family connections weren't as strong as they could have been. Our family "safety net" was stretched too thin and had too many holes in it. Our love for Libby and our concern for her mental health never diminished, but we were scattered around the country. I was in Maryland, her mother in Florida, Graham in North

Carolina, and Will in Tennessee. Each of us tried to stay in touch with Libby and with each other, but none of us had a complete picture of Libby – her emotional state, relationships, living arrangements, finances, legal problems and other significant stressors. We each had only a few pieces of the puzzle, and we didn't communicate as frequently or as well as we could have.

Speaking for myself, I wish that I had made more trips to Florida and insisted on seeing Libby more often. I'm not sure exactly what I would have been able to accomplish, but I might have gained a better, more complete understanding of her situation and been able to help her find solutions to some of her problems. I also wish I had asked more probing questions when I did talk with her and been more skeptical of some of her responses.

Finally, although my conversations with Mary, Mike, Jordan, Graham and Will brought back painful memories of Libby's struggles with depression, we also found ourselves remembering many of the good times and many of her wonderful qualities. I believe it is very important that we don't forget these. While I still feel the loss and grieve every single day for Libby, I also remind myself to be grateful for the time I did have with her. She brought so much joy and meaning into my life. I can honestly say that I was truly blessed to have this wonderful daughter in my life for thirty-six years, and I still smile when I think of the many good times we had together and the love she shared with me and so many others.

CHAPTER 4

RECOGNIZING AND RESPONDING TO DEPRESSION

While it is clear that depression is a painful and potentially lethal illness, there is good news about depression that needs to be shared – that it is a highly treatable condition. Most individuals can be successfully treated for depression. However, far too many people who suffer from depression fail to receive effective treatment. Often the failure to be treated is because of one or more of the following obstacles:

⇨ Failure to recognize the symptoms of depression
⇨ Stigma
⇨ Pessimism and misconceptions about treatment

Before reviewing treatments for depression, I think it's helpful to understand these obstacles and what can be done to overcome them.

W. DANIEL HALE, PhD

Failure to recognize the symptoms of depression

One of the barriers that can interfere with individuals receiving the treatment they need is that they fail to recognize they are depressed. They may know that something is wrong, but they don't realize that what they are going through is a serious illness. That is why it's important to be able to recognize the symptoms of depression:

⇨ *Depressed mood with overwhelming feelings of sadness and grief* — Depressed individuals usually report being profoundly and persistently sad or unhappy, although they may not readily share this with others. Unless they are tearful or their facial expression suggests sadness, their depressed mood may go unnoticed – even by family and friends. In adolescents, irritability is often seen instead of sadness.

⇨ *Loss of interest and pleasure in activities formerly enjoyed* — People with depression typically lose the ability to enjoy their work, their leisure activities and even their interactions with family and friends. While it's not uncommon to fail to detect a person's depressed mood, this symptom is easier to notice because it usually leads to observable changes in behavior. Depressed individuals often stop participating in activities they previously enjoyed or – if they do continue the activities – show little enthusiasm for them. Adolescents who are depressed often drop out of usual activities (e.g., sports, musical groups, social clubs) and withdraw from friends.

⇨ *Noticeable changes in appetite and weight (significant weight loss or gain)* — Although some people who are depressed turn to food for comfort or develop cravings for high calorie foods that result in weight gain, many depressed individuals lose weight because food has lost its appeal. And, often times, they don't have the energy to prepare something to eat or to go out to a restaurant for a healthy meal.

⇨ *Insomnia, early morning waking or oversleeping* — Depression often brings with it a significant change in sleep patterns. Some people sleep more when they are depressed, but often seriously depressed individuals have trouble getting a full night of restful, restorative sleep. Instead, they find themselves having difficulty falling asleep, or they wake up in the middle of the night or earlier than usual and have trouble going back to sleep.

⇨ *Being physically slowed down or restlessness* — When depressed persons move or talk, they often do so more slowly than normal. They also may find that they think more slowly, thus taking more time to respond to questions or having more difficulty engaging in conversations with others. It's also possible that they experience restlessness and agitation, finding that they can't sit or stand still and instead spend much of their time pacing back and forth.

⇨ *Decreased energy or fatigue* — When someone is depressed, they often have trouble finding the strength and energy to perform tasks that they previously could do effortlessly. The smallest task or briefest activity can seem overwhelming. They report being constantly tired, even when they haven't been exerting themselves physically.

⇨ *Feelings of worthlessness, guilt or hopelessness* — Depressed individuals often talk about how they feel like a fraud or an imposter. They believe they have been fooling people and don't deserve any of the positive recognition or good things they have received. Some talk about how they feel responsible for or guilty about many of the bad events that are happening in their life. They may blame themselves for things that are not their responsibility or greatly exaggerate their failures. What makes this even worse is that these negative thoughts play on a constant loop in their head. Depressed adolescents, feeling worthless or hopeless, may give up on plans to attend college or even decide to drop out of school.

⇨ *Difficulty concentrating or thinking, indecisiveness* — A depressed person often reports difficulty thinking or concentrating. Someone who enjoyed reading may have trouble staying focused for more than a paragraph or two at a time. Their mind will wander off, focusing instead on negative experiences or expectations. They also may have difficulty making decisions that previously would have been easy to make. Or they may find themselves forgetting things. One concern about memory problems associated with depression – especially if they occur in an older person – is that they may be mistakenly seen as evidence of dementia. For adolescents, problems with concentration often lead to a decline in academic performance and lower grades.

⇨ *Recurrent thoughts of death or suicide* — Along with impaired thinking, the emotional pain and hopelessness of depression can leave some people feeling that their only escape is death. Or they may believe that others would be better off if they were dead. Some actively think about ways they could hasten their death, while others simply wish that death could come sooner.

A diagnosis of major depression is given when a person has experienced five or more of these symptoms every day or almost every day during a two-week period, with at least one of the symptoms being depressed mood or loss of interest or pleasure in activities previously enjoyed. However, if you have fewer than five symptoms but they are causing you emotional distress and impacting your relationships, work and daily responsibilities, it's still a good idea to talk to your health care provider or a mental health professional.

Another mood disorder in which a person experiences episodes of depression is bipolar disorder (also known as manic-depressive disorder). In addition to depression, the person experiences periods of mania or hypomania. The manic episodes are characterized by periods of abnormally and persistently elevated or irritable mood, along with excessive activity. These episodes are severe enough to cause significant problems at work and at home. Hypomanic episodes involve milder manic symptoms. It is important that individuals who experience either mania or hypomania along with their depression share this information with their health care provider because it will help determine the appropriate treatment. More information about bipolar disorder can be found on websites for the National Institute of Mental Health and the Depression and Bipolar Support Alliance (listed along with other resources in Chapter 7).

Stigma

Most people don't hesitate to discuss common medical conditions, such as hypertension or diabetes, with family and friends. In fact, they would probably have no problem sharing their latest blood pressure reading or A1C level, and they wouldn't mind mentioning the health professional who is providing their care. Unfortunately, often the same is not true when it comes to depression. Many people who suffer from depression do not feel comfortable talking about what they are experiencing because they are afraid that others will not view depression the same way they view other medical conditions. They worry that instead of being understood and supported, they might be criticized for being weak or for failing to appreciate just how fortunate they are.

In addition to feeling misunderstood or criticized for being depressed, there's also the fear that their friends might think less of them or that their opportunities for career advancement might be limited if their supervisor or co-workers learn of their depression.

Of particular concern to me is that members of religious congregations frequently choose not to reach out to clergy or fellow congregants when they are depressed. They fear that they will be told that the reason they are depressed is because of their sinfulness or that their faith is not strong enough, and that the only advice they would receive is to pray more.

Also, it's not unusual to find that individuals suffering from depression internalize some of the negative perceptions of depression. I have to confess that this was true of me. Despite my training as a psychologist, my belief that depression should be viewed as a medical condition, and my recognition that I needed professional care, there were times when I blamed myself. I had been strong enough to overcome other serious challenges in my life, so why couldn't I find the strength to overcome my depression?

What I needed to remember – and what all of us who experience depression need to understand and remember – is that depression is a medical condition. There is no reason for us to feel ashamed or embarrassed. Having said that, I'm not recommending that we speak openly about our depression with everyone. Rather, I believe we should share what we are experiencing with trusted health care providers and with family members or friends who care about us and want to understand what they can do to help.

Pessimism and misconceptions about treatment

Another barrier to treatment is the sense of hopelessness that is a central element of depression. Even if people recognize that they are depressed and understand there is no reason to be embarrassed about their illness, they still may not seek treatment because they believe there is nothing that can be done to help them. Their persistent pessimism may cause them to feel that they are trapped in a permanent state of depression, or they may believe that while treatment for depression has worked for others, it will not work for them.

Misconceptions about treatment could also serve as a barrier. People may believe that the only treatments available for depression are lengthy and extremely expensive. This is why it is so important that we understand – and regularly remind ourselves and others – that there are effective treatments. It might take time to find the right treatment, but almost all individuals suffering from depression – even severe forms – will be able to benefit from treatment.

TREATMENT STRATEGIES AND OPTIONS

If, after reviewing the symptoms listed at the beginning of this chapter, you think you might be depressed, you should schedule an appointment with your primary health care provider or a mental health professional (psychiatrist, psychologist, clinical social worker or mental health counselor) as soon as possible. One of the benefits of going to your primary health care provider first is that there are medications and medical conditions (e.g., thyroid disorders, electrolyte abnormalities, vitamin deficiencies) that can produce symptoms similar to those of depression. To rule these out, your provider may conduct a physical exam or run some lab tests.

Your provider also will ask detailed questions about your symptoms. To make your medical visit as easy and productive as possible, it will be helpful if you take detailed notes about what you have been experiencing to your appointment. The information should include:

⇨ A list of the symptoms you have been experiencing, including their severity. Be as specific as you can. When did they begin? If they are not constant, then at what times or in what situations do they occur? What makes them improve or become worse? Have you ever had these symptoms before? If so, how long ago and how were they treated? How are these symptoms affecting your day-to-day life?

⇨ A special note about any possible symptoms of mania (e.g., decreased need for sleep, being more talkative than usual, feeling that your thoughts are racing, having exceedingly high activity levels, thinking you can do a lot of things at once) or hypomania (symptoms similar to those of mania but less severe and less likely to impair relationships or work).

⇨ Any remedies you have already tried. Have you taken any over-the-counter medications? Have you changed your diet or any of your habits in an attempt to address the problem? If so, did your efforts help?

⇨ A list of medications, including nonprescription medications and nutritional supplements. One of the best ways to provide this information is for you to take all your medications with you to your appointment. Also mention any treatments you are receiving that may not be strictly medical (e.g., acupuncture, chiropractic care, homeopathic care).

⇨ Any significant changes in your life recently (e.g., illness or death of a loved one, difficulties in relationships with family or friends, new living arrangements, change in finances, new responsibilities at home or at work or at your place of worship, change in your ability to handle household matters).

One more step you should consider as you prepare for your medical visit is to ask a family member or friend to go with you. If you think that it might be difficult for you to present all the information that needs to be shared, to ask important questions or to remember exactly what is recommended, then ask someone to accompany you to your appointment.

Some primary care providers feel comfortable diagnosing and treating depression, while others may want to refer you to a psychiatrist or other mental health professional after ruling out other medical conditions. If your provider concludes you are depressed and feels comfortable treating depression, you may be given a prescription for an antidepressant medication. General information about antidepressant medications is provided later in this chapter, but be sure you have enough information about the specific medication you have been prescribed before you leave your appointment. Some of the questions you should ask are:

⇨   What are the expected benefits of the medication?
⇨   How long will it take for me to notice the benefits?
⇨   How should it be taken and how often?
⇨   Will this medication interfere with any of my other medications?
⇨   What are the side effects of the medication? What should I do if I experience them?

Be sure to write down the answers to these questions and review your notes with your provider before you leave. If there is any reason why you might not be able to take the medication you have been prescribed, do not hesitate to mention this to your provider. Doctors and other health care providers understand and appreciate the fact that the latest and best medication for a medical condition is of no value if it is not taken as prescribed. If the cost of the medication is the obstacle, explain this to your provider. Often, a less expensive alternative with similar benefits is available.

It's also possible that your primary health care provider will recommend psychotherapy with a mental health professional (psychologist, clinical social worker or mental health counselor) instead of or in addition to medication. If your provider doesn't suggest that you see a psychotherapist but you feel that it would be helpful to talk with someone, ask for a referral or recommendation. For most people suffering from depression, the combination of medication and psychotherapy is best. More information about psychotherapy is provided later in this chapter.

It's important to note that although more than half of all mental health care is delivered in the primary care setting, some providers may feel more comfortable referring you to a mental health professional for treatment, especially if there is uncertainty about the diagnosis, concern about the severity of the symptoms, the presence of other psychiatric conditions or significant risk for suicide. Most likely, you will be referred to a psychiatrist, a physician who specializes in mental disorders and can prescribe medications. Psychiatrists also are trained in psychotherapy, but many limit their practice to medical treatments and prefer to refer to other mental health professionals if they believe a patient would benefit from psychotherapy.

If you are referred to a psychiatrist, you may encounter difficulty scheduling an appointment within a few days or even weeks due to a shortage of psychiatrists in many communities. If you find that the first appointment you can schedule is several weeks away and you feel you need professional care before then, you can ask for a referral to a non-medical mental health professional who has experience treating depression. Many psychologists, clinical social workers and mental health counselors have the experience and expertise to treat mood disorders and can help you manage your depression until you can see a psychiatrist.

If you choose to go directly to a non-medical mental health professional for treatment of your depression, they may recommend that you also see your primary care provider so that other potential causes of depression symptoms can be ruled out. It's also possible that your therapist will encourage you to talk to a psychiatrist or your primary care provider about including medication as part of your treatment.

Antidepressant Medications

Antidepressant medications can be effective in relieving the painful symptoms of depression and helping restore you to your normal level of functioning, but it's important to have an understanding of how these medications are used and what to expect.

Antidepressants do not provide immediate relief. While you may feel a modest improvement in your mood within the first couple of weeks, it can take four to eight weeks for a significant therapeutic benefit to be felt. During this period, it is important that you take the medication exactly as prescribed, stay in regular contact with your health care provider, and report any unpleasant side effects or other reasons why you are concerned about the drug (e.g., cost). Fortunately, there are several types of antidepressants and a number of options within each class. Your provider likely can find another option if a side effect or the cost of the medication is a problem. If side effects are not a problem but you're feeling little or no improvement after several weeks, your provider likely will want to adjust the dosage or substitute another type of antidepressant. This shouldn't be surprising or discouraging. It's not unusual for it to take some time to find the right medication and the right dose. Because this could take several weeks or even longer, it's often helpful to be working with a psychotherapist at the same time.

Once you have experienced relief from all your symptoms, you will need to talk with your provider about exactly when and how the medication should be discontinued. Although patients are often tempted to discontinue antidepressants as soon as they feel they have recovered, it is generally recommended that you continue taking the medication for another six to twelve months. Doing so reduces the risk of depression returning. And when you do discontinue the medication, you shouldn't do it abruptly. You will need to work closely with your provider to slowly and safely reduce the dose.

Additional, up-to-date information on antidepressant medications can be found on websites for the National Institute of Mental Health and MedlinePlus (listed along with other resources in Chapter 7).

Psychotherapy

Psychotherapy, or what is often referred to as "talk therapy," has been found to be an effective treatment for mild to moderate forms of depression and is often used in combination with medication. There are several types of psychotherapy, but all involve a collaborative and confidential relationship with a mental health professional. Sessions are typically 45

– 50 minutes in length and scheduled once a week; however, more frequent sessions may be advisable at the beginning of therapy or during an especially difficult period.

The confidential nature of the relationship is essential, allowing patients to speak openly about their thoughts, feelings and experiences without fear of being judged or concerns about the information being shared with anyone else. Therapists are required by both their professional ethics and the law to maintain this confidentiality unless they believe there is an immediate threat to the safety of the patient or other persons, or if they learn of the abuse, exploitation or neglect of children, the elderly or people with disabilities.

Two forms of psychotherapy for which there is solid evidence of their effectiveness in the treatment of depression are cognitive behavioral therapy (CBT) and interpersonal therapy (IPT). Both are generally considered short-term therapies – ranging from about five to twenty sessions. Therapists may combine elements of CBT with elements of IPT or other approaches. This is often referred to as "eclectic therapy."

The objective of cognitive behavioral therapy is to help people identify and then modify unhealthy, negative thoughts and behaviors. Although past experiences are not ignored, greater emphasis is placed on the present – the beliefs and behaviors that are contributing to and maintaining the depression. In addition to using therapy sessions to examine and modify negative beliefs, some of the time may be devoted to developing a schedule of mood- and confidence-enhancing activities that can be carried out between sessions.

Interpersonal therapy is a short-term therapy that is especially effective when a person's depression is associated with a significant loss (e.g., death of a loved one, divorce), troubled relationships or being faced with new, unfamiliar relationships and responsibilities. It can help patients gain a better understanding of interpersonal issues, work through the emotions associated with these issues, and develop skills to meet new challenges.

Whatever the therapeutic approach, a strong, collaborative relationship between you and your therapist is absolutely critical. You need to feel comfortable talking openly and honestly about your thoughts and feelings. One place to start your search for a psychotherapist is with your primary care provider or one of your other health providers. Ask if they know of a psychologist, clinical social worker or mental health counselor with experience treating depression. Another option available to many individuals is their employer's Employee Assistance Program (EAP). These programs typically provide free and confidential assessments, short-term counseling, and referrals. Trusted family members, friends and members of the clergy also may be able to provide a recommendation. Searching online is another option. Most therapists have websites that provide information about their education, professional credentials and areas of expertise. They also may include how long they have been in practice, office hours, fees and whether or not they accept insurance.

When you first meet with a psychotherapist, don't hesitate to ask any questions, including questions about the therapist's training, professional license, certifications, experience, fees and confidentiality. Another concern for some people is how their religious beliefs and practices are viewed by mental health professionals. If you have this concern, ask the therapist. Therapists and patients don't have to share the same faith, but it is important for therapists to respect and be sensitive to their patients' religious beliefs and practices.

While you shouldn't expect psychotherapy to produce instant results, you should expect to feel comfortable with your therapist and confident that the two of you can work in partnership. If you don't, then talk to your therapist about what seems to be missing in the relationship. Perhaps a different approach would help. If this doesn't seem possible or prove beneficial, then it's reasonable to consider switching to a different therapist.

MY TREATMENT EXPERIENCE

When I experienced my first episode of depression, I sought the help of both my primary care physician and a psychologist. My physician, who had provided my medical care for almost a decade and knew me well, prescribed an antidepressant. Within six weeks, it restored my appetite and energy and helped me sleep well. It had a couple side effects that were initially bothersome, but they were clearly outweighed by the benefits of the medication and diminished over time.

While the medication was helping with the physical symptoms of depression, my psychologist helped me with other aspects. He took an eclectic approach, using cognitive behavioral therapy to address my negative beliefs and behaviors and interpersonal therapy to work on the challenges I was facing as a recently divorced father of three young children.

One of the negative beliefs that was having a far-reaching impact on my life concerned my career. I had become convinced that I was an absolutely awful professor and that my students must be terribly disappointed in me. This belief was so powerful that I dreaded going to campus each day. My therapist listened closely and empathetically to what I was saying and then gently and skillfully challenged this belief. He helped me see how I was ignoring evidence that students might be enjoying my classes and greatly exaggerating anything that was the least bit negative. He also gave me a homework assignment – I was to ask my students to anonymously complete course evaluations. When I did, I found that my current students, just like students in earlier years when I felt good about myself and my classes, gave my courses very positive evaluations. This helped me appreciate just how distorted and inaccurate some of my core beliefs about myself were. With my psychologist's help, I was able to examine and gradually alter those beliefs, which gave me greater confidence and led to positive changes in my behavior.

I also needed help dealing with the difficult relationship transitions I was experiencing. I had been married for eighteen years and shared parenting duties with my wife for twelve of those years. Now, I was living by myself half of the time and parenting three children on my own the rest of the time. I had doubts about my ability to handle some of these new responsibilities and concerns about what the failure of my marriage meant with respect to any future relationships. This is where the interpersonal therapy my psychologist incorporated into our sessions was beneficial. It helped me understand and work through some of the issues and emotions associated with the demise of my marriage. The therapy also helped me develop effective strategies and skills as I faced new relationship challenges.

After being symptom-free for six months, my physician, psychologist and I decided that it was safe for me to gradually discontinue the antidepressant medication and psychotherapy. I felt confident that my depressive episode was well behind me – and I was right. For the next seventeen years, I was free of depression. That isn't to say that life wasn't difficult at times and that I never felt sad, but I certainly never experienced the painful, debilitating symptoms of a major depression.

My treatment experience was somewhat different when I suffered my second episode of depression – the one that came during a period of my life when everything seemed to be going so well. My longtime primary care provider was out of the country on a lengthy vacation, so I was referred by his office to another physician who prescribed one of the newer medications for depression. This drug did not have the desired effect. In fact, it increased my anxiety. He switched me to another antidepressant medication, but this also brought on anxiety. At that point, I felt I needed a specialist and was able to schedule an appointment with a psychiatrist. After a careful, detailed evaluation, she prescribed another antidepressant from a different class of drugs. One of the reasons she chose this medication was because of its sedating effect, something I felt I needed since one of the worst symptoms I was experiencing was severe sleep disturbance. Thankfully, this medication worked as we hoped it would. It gradually, gently improved my moods, restored my energy, and guaranteed that I could get a restful sleep each night. I also found it helpful to schedule a few sessions with the psychologist during this period as I struggled with self-doubts that had arisen again. Using a blend of cognitive behavioral therapy and interpersonal therapy, he helped me regain my confidence and re-establish healthy work and interpersonal routines.

I then faced an important decision. How long should I stay on the medication? While it's generally recommended that you stay on an antidepressant for at least six to twelve months after all symptoms are gone, there are times that it is advisable to stay on the medication even longer, perhaps indefinitely. My psychiatrist and I decided that this was the best course for me. It's now been fourteen years since I started on this particular antidepressant. During this time, I have experienced several extremely stressful events and the painful loss of my oldest daughter, but I have been able to manage these challenges without sinking into a serious depression. Had I not remained on my medication, I'm not sure how I would have handled these life events or if I would have returned to a depressive state. That being said, I believe my decision to stay on the antidepressant has been the right decision for me. My mental health is equally – if not more – important than my physical health.

Just as I take a statin every night to control my cholesterol and reduce the risk of a heart attack or stroke, I take an antidepressant every night to help with my mood and to reduce the risk of another painful episode of depression.

CHAPTER 5

CARING FOR A LOVED ONE

Caring for a loved one who is depressed can be challenging. You may find yourself experiencing confusion, frustration, and a sense of helplessness. Some of the things depressed individuals say and do can be difficult to understand, and even hurtful. It's hard not to take it personally when your loved one no longer seems to enjoy being with you or appreciate your attempts to be helpful and supportive. You may find yourself bewildered by changes in their attitude and behavior. Why would someone who has always been active and hardworking no longer want to go to work? Why would a teenager who has been successful academically and has plenty of friends no longer want to go to school? How can a person who has so much to look forward to have such a bleak view of life and the future? And young children who have a parent suffering with depression may find it especially difficult to understand why their parent is no longer as attentive or affectionate.

Because depression can have a serious, far-reaching impact on a person's attitudes, thoughts and behaviors, it's important for family members and friends to educate themselves as much as they can about this condition. You need to be able to recognize the symptoms of depression, understand the treatments and learn what you can say and do to aid in your loved one's recovery. While you can't be expected to "fix" someone who is depressed, you can play a crucial role by offering understanding and support.

PURSUING TREATMENT

The most important thing you can do for a family member or friend who is showing signs of depression is to encourage them to seek professional help. If your loved one has not acknowledged being depressed or recognized the need for treatment, you can begin by sharing what you have observed and why you are concerned. Describe the changes in behavior or attitude you have noticed. Explain why you think these changes could be signs of depression and why you believe it would be wise for them to schedule an appointment with their primary care provider or a mental health professional. As you do this, make sure your loved one understands that you are not being critical or judgmental – that your only reason for expressing concern is because you want to help. Emphasize that you view depression as a medical condition, not as a personal weakness or failure. There is no reason for anyone who has depression to feel embarrassed or ashamed.

It can be difficult to persuade some people who are depressed to seek professional care, even if they are not embarrassed about being depressed. One reason is the sense of pessimism that typically accompanies this condition. Depressed individuals often feel their situation is hopeless – that there is nothing that can help them get better.

Another reason is that depression saps a person's energy. Even if depressed individuals acknowledge that there might be effective treatments for depression, many simply don't have the energy to research treatment options or locate possible providers. This is where family and friends can play an important role. By learning enough basic information about treatments for depression, you can assure your loved one – with confidence – that there is help for their condition. You may also want to offer to help them schedule an appointment with their primary care provider or search for a mental health professional.

Don't be surprised if it takes more than one conversation to convince your loved one to seek the care of a health professional. That's why it's important for you to stay in regular contact and to continue to share your concerns and offer assistance. If your loved one continues to express reluctance about seeing a health professional, then you may want to say something like, "I understand that you feel you don't need to talk with a health professional about what you're experiencing, but *I* would feel much better if you did. Please, just do it for me."

If you are successful in persuading your loved one to seek professional care, then you can offer to assist them as they prepare for the appointment. You can help them construct a list of symptoms along with any information about current circumstances or recent developments in their life. You also can offer to accompany them to their appointment.

One important piece of information about depression that family members and friends need to understand is that the treatments for depression take time – often as long as six to eight weeks. It's easy for depressed individuals to get discouraged when they don't see a difference right away. They may stop taking their medication or skip appointments with their therapist. A valuable role you can play is to continue encouraging your loved one to stick with their treatment plan.

OFFERING SUPPORT AND ENCOURAGEMENT

Since treatments can take a number of weeks to be effective, there is a need for family and friends to stay in regular contact and to continue offering their love, support and encouragement. Even if a person is fortunate enough to see a therapist for an hour every week, there are still one hundred and sixty-seven other hours in the week. The concern, love, understanding and companionship offered by family and friends during these hours are invaluable.

> The concern, love, understanding and companionship offered by family and friends during these hours are invaluable.

It's important to emphasize to your loved one that you sincerely want to be of help. When you offer support, it's not enough to say, "Please call me if there is anything I can do to help." Depressed individuals often don't feel worthy of someone else's time and attention. They may not reach out to you or others for assistance, so you may need to take the initiative.

When I tell a friend who is depressed that I want to stay in touch and help, I'm frequently told, "You don't have to do that." My response is, "I know I don't have to, but I *want* to. I care about you and I want to be there for you during this difficult time." I then follow up with regular calls or visits, which are always appreciated.

One of the things that was most helpful to me the first time I was seriously depressed was having a fellow faculty member insist on taking me to lunch every Friday. I was feeling so bad about myself that I didn't think I deserved the time and attention of this distinguished professor, but he wouldn't take "no" for an answer. During our lunches, he didn't offer advice or tell me that I needed to "get over" my depression. Instead, he listened patiently as I talked about my feelings and how everything seemed hopeless. He never dismissed or tried to minimize what I was feel-ing, but he found ways to slip into our conversations little reminders of how I had been successful and how I was liked and respected by colleagues and students. He also expressed confidence that I would recover. Although I didn't feel optimistic, I still found it reassuring that he was. And he always conveyed – in words and actions – that he genuinely cared about me.

When I experienced my second episode, I was fortunate to have my wife, Kim, looking out for me. One of the most valuable things she did was to find a psychiatrist to help with medication when the first antidepressants prescribed to me were not working. There were also things she did almost every day that helped carry me through this emotionally painful period. Kim called me regularly to see how I was feeling and to assure me that she loved me. She also gently, but firmly, insisted that we continue our nightly walks around the neighborhood with our dogs, even though I didn't feel like I had the energy. Additionally, she took over my household responsibilities whenever I felt overwhelmed. Through all of this, she never made me feel guilty or that I was a burden for her, and she regularly reminded me that she was certain I would recover from this episode – just as I had recovered from the earlier episode.

I heard many similar stories when a colleague and I surveyed individuals who had experienced a serious depression. We asked what their families and friends had done that was most helpful, and this is what they said:

"They called regularly to see how I was doing."

"They came over and spent time with me."

"Sometimes they just sat quietly and patiently with me."

"They listened carefully to what I said. They wanted to understand what I was going through"

"They gently pushed me to go for walks with them or on brief shopping trips."

"They expressed a quiet but deep confidence that with time and treatment I would get better."

"They told me how much they cared for me. That they loved me."

"They helped with some of my tasks when I was feeling overwhelmed."

"They reminded me of my positive qualities and the good things I had accomplished."

"They helped me get back into a healthy routine."

We also asked about some of the things people said that were not helpful. Almost everyone we asked had at least one good example of what *not* to say. Among the examples given were:

"They told me to 'snap out of it' or 'get over it.'"

"They said I should remember how fortunate I was – that there were others who had it much worse."

"They told me to just think positive thoughts."

"They assured me that all I needed to do was to pray more."

RECOGNIZING THE RISK OF SUICIDE

Individuals with depression are at a higher risk of suicide than those without depression. It's important to be able to recognize the warning signs and to know what you should say or do if someone you know appears to be suicidal.

The National Institute of Mental Health lists the following as signs that someone may be thinking about suicide:

⇨ Talking about wanting to die or wanting to kill themselves

⇨ Talking about feeling empty, hopeless or having no reason to live

⇨ Planning or looking for a way to kill themselves, such as searching online, stockpiling pills or newly acquiring potentially lethal items (e.g., firearms, ropes)

⇨ Talking about great guilt or shame

⇨ Talking about feeling trapped or feeling that there are no solutions

⇨ Feeling unbearable pain, both physical or emotional

⇨ Talking about being a burden to others

⇨ Using alcohol or drugs more often

⇨ Acting anxious or agitated

⇨ Withdrawing from family and friends

⇨ Changing eating and/or sleeping habits

⇨ Showing rage or talking about seeking revenge

⇨ Taking risks that could lead to death, such as reckless driving

⇨ Talking or thinking about death often

⇨ Displaying extreme mood swings, suddenly changing from very sad to very calm or happy

⇨ Giving away important possessions

⇨ Saying goodbye to friends and family

⇨ Putting affairs in order, making a will

If you see or hear any of these warning signs, take them seriously. Share your concern with the person, and don't be reluctant to ask if they are thinking of harming themselves. You will not be putting the idea into their head.

If you believe that there is an immediate risk of suicide, do not leave the person alone. You can call 911 or the National Suicide Prevention Lifeline at 1-800-273-TALK (1-800-273-8255), or take the person to a hospital emergency department or your local psychiatric crisis center.

If you find that there is not an immediate risk of suicide but you remain concerned about what you have seen or heard, you can share your concern with the person's health care provider and family members. You can also take steps to keep the person's environment safer by removing or locking up items that could be used in a suicide attempt, such as firearms, medications or ropes. If your loved one is talking about the appeal of death – either by suicide or natural causes – be open with your feelings. Express your affection. Let the person know how much you love them and how much you would miss them if they were to die.

FINDING TIME FOR SELF-CARE

It's not easy to live with someone who is seriously depressed. In many respects, it's like living with a different person. So much about the individual you have known and enjoyed seems to have disappeared. And it's not unusual to feel personally rejected when your loved one talks about how absolutely nothing in life is good and that there is nothing that makes life worth living. You may feel like saying, "But what about me?" It can be especially painful when depression affects intimate relationships, as it often does. It's also easy for family members to blame themselves for the problems their loved one is experiencing, even though they are doing their best to support that person. This is why it is important for people who are living with or caring for depressed individuals to make a special effort to also care for themselves.

One of the most valuable things you can do is to develop your own support system. You shouldn't try to go through the experience of caring for a loved one for what could be a lengthy period of time by yourself. Major depressive episodes can last, on average, more than six months. This is a time to reach out to friends for help. And it's particularly important to have someone to talk to about how your loved one's depression is impacting you. There needs to be someone who can help you with a "reality check" when your loved one is saying or doing hurtful things. Most often, it's the depression that is responsible for these words and actions, and it's helpful to have someone who understands this and can encourage you not to take it personally. This could be a close, trusted friend, a clergyperson or a mental health professional. When you talk with this person, you don't need to share everything your loved one is saying or doing. You certainly don't want to betray confidences. Instead, focus on what you're feeling and how your loved one's depression is affecting you.

It's also important to maintain a healthy lifestyle. Make sure you set aside time for yourself as much as possible and continue with some of the activities you find rewarding and renewing. Remember, if you don't take good care of yourself, you're not going to be able to take good care of your loved one.

CHAPTER 6

MINISTERING TO THE VULNERABLE AMONG US

One of the principal teachings of my faith is our responsibility to care for the most vulnerable among us. Growing up, that often meant volunteering at a program for the hungry and homeless in our community, visiting frail elderly in nursing homes, or working with severely disabled children at the state hospital. Later, there were opportunities to reach out to those in the community who were suffering from discrimination and extreme poverty. For me, the focus on caring for the vulnerable and suffering always meant reaching beyond the walls of the church. It didn't occur to me to also look inside the church. It wasn't until I began working with the seriously depressed that I realized many of the individuals experiencing the greatest sense of vulnerability and despair are sitting in our church pews on Sunday mornings, suffering in silence. Later, I would be one of those individuals – feeling more vulnerable and desperate than I had ever imagined.

> The need for churches and other faith communities to reach out and care for those suffering with depression has never been greater.

The need for churches and other faith communities to reach out and care for those suffering with depression has never been greater. Depression is now recognized as one of our most serious public health concerns. Every year, more than ten percent of adults experience a major depressive episode. Furthermore, depression is the major risk factor for suicide, now one of the top ten leading causes of death. And we also know that depression is a significant risk factor for substance abuse – another of our most serious public health concerns.

While we might want to believe that our religious faith can protect us from depression and suicide, we know that's not true. We have heard too many stories of religious leaders and members of deeply religious families who have suffered from depression and taken their own lives. We need to recognize that depression doesn't discriminate. It is found among the young and old, the religious and nonreligious, and all ethnic and racial groups.

The challenge for us as people of faith is to create communities where individuals experiencing the crippling pain and despair of depression can feel safe turning to their clergy and fellow congregants. A place where they are confident they will be understood and supported, and not judged. This starts by bringing the topic of depression out of the darkness and into the light. We must begin talking about it more openly – in our youth groups, adult classes, older adult programs and even from the pulpit.

One of the key points we need to emphasize is that clinical depression is not the same as the sadness or blues we all experience from time to time. It is a serious illness that can be life limiting and even life threatening. But we also need to stress the good news about depression – that it is a treatable illness, and that there is hope for those who suffer from it. These are the messages that we need to share throughout our congregations and beyond.

We can begin by providing educational materials about depression at worship services and other congregational gatherings. This will help people recognize what depression looks like and understand the tremendous impact it can have on individuals. Additionally, we can provide encouragement and guidance about where to turn for help if individuals believe they or a loved one might be depressed. This includes basic information about treatment options, local resources and when to consult with their family physician or a mental health professional.

We also can organize special programs on depression following our worship services or as part of other congregational gatherings. These programs can include more extensive educational materials and speakers who can present important perspectives on depression. We can invite representatives from organizations that advocate on behalf of those with depression and other mental health conditions (e.g., National Alliance on Mental Illness/NAMI, Mental Health America); mental health professionals who can speak about diagnosis and treatment; and individuals who have suffered with depression and are willing to share their personal experiences. (One source for such speakers is the "In Our Own Voice" program offered by many NAMI affiliates.) We also can offer groups, or connect people to groups in the community, where those who are directly or indirectly impacted by depression can share their stories and talk with others who are facing similar challenges.

It's often helpful to schedule these programs to coincide with national health awareness campaigns. For example, May is designated as Mental Health Month, and each year national organizations (e.g., NAMI, Mental Health America and the National Institute of Mental Health) sponsor a number of activities to increase awareness. Other options are July, which is designated as Minority Mental Health Month, and October, which is Depression Awareness Month.

As we plan congregational programs, we need to be aware that some people affected by depression may not feel comfortable attending a program that is focused exclusively on depression. They may want to keep their interest in the topic a private matter. I believe it is important to recognize and respect their wishes; however, they are often the ones with the greatest need for information. One way we can handle this is to have the program be part of a regularly scheduled group meeting or activity where people would be attending regardless of the topic. Another option is to have the program focused more broadly, perhaps covering stress as well as depression. Most people have no problem acknowledging that they experience stress and wouldn't hesitate to attend a program on the topic.

This brings us to the serious issue of stigma. Unfortunately, too many people still have a negative association when it comes to depression. They don't view it the same way they view other common medical conditions, such as diabetes or heart disease. Instead, they believe depression is a reflection of personal weakness, a character defect or lack of faith. Such beliefs can keep people from receiving the information, care and support they need. I believe that it's important for all of us – especially our religious leaders – to directly and explicitly confront the issue of stigma. We need to let people of faith know that they should not be embarrassed or ashamed if they suffer from depression, and that they should not hesitate to seek professional care, just as they would if they had diabetes or heart disease.

Part of the approach to battling stigma among people of faith can be sharing examples from the Bible of major figures who suffered with depression. Many find their stories to be reassuring. Dr. Pat Fosarelli, MD, a theologian, physician and lay minister who teaches spirituality and practical theology at St. Mary's Ecumenical Institute in Baltimore, has shared some of the scripture passages she has found helpful when ministering to individuals suffering with depression.

⇨ The prophet Elijah prayed for death, "This is enough, O Lord. Take my life…" (1 Kings 19: 4)

⇨ In a long prayer, the prophet Jeremiah prayed, "Cursed be the day on which I was born!" (Jeremiah 20: 14) and "Why did I come forth from the womb to see sorrow and pain, to end my days in shame?" (Jeremiah 20: 18)

⇨ The prophet Jonah prayed for death, "Please take my life from me, for it is better for me to die than to live." (Jonah 4: 3) and "I would be better off dead than alive." (Jonah 4: 8)

⇨ After the shame of his adulterous affair with Bathsheba, the murder of her husband, and the birth of the child of Bathsheba and King David, he could not eat and remained lying on the ground in sackcloth. (2 Samuel 12: 16-17)

⇨ After losing his family and his wealth, Job cried out, "Sighing comes more readily to me than food, and my groans well forth like water. For what I fear overtakes me, and what I shrink from comes upon me. I have no peace nor ease. I have no rest, for trouble comes." (Job 3: 24-26)

⇨ Hannah is so distraught because she cannot have a child that her distress is perceived as drunkenness (1 Samuel 1: 13-16); she weeps and refuses to eat. (1 Samuel 1:7)

⇨ The Psalms have many references to feeling abandoned by God; perhaps the most poignant is the opening of Psalm 22: "My God, my God, why have you abandoned me? Why so far from my call for help, from my cries of anguish? My God, I call by day, but you do not answer; by night, and I have no relief."

While educating our congregations about depression and battling stigma are certainly important, I believe we can do more. We can be prepared and empowered to act on what we have learned, especially when our words and actions have the potential to literally save lives. When we notice changes in a person's mood, attitude or behavior that could be signs of depression (e.g., not attending worship services or other activities they previously enjoyed, appearing more tired than usual, expressing a sense of hopelessness), we can take the initiative to discreetly share with them what we have observed and express our concern. When we do, we may discover that the changes we have noticed are not due to depression. Perhaps we will find that they are the result of changes in their work schedule or family responsibilities and that there is no reason to be concerned. But if it turns out that our concerns are justified – that they are depressed – we can play a critical role by offering the support, encouragement and assistance that can help them start on the path to recovery.

Meaningful support begins by listening attentively and patiently as they share what they are experiencing. The words we offer in response need to not only reflect our love and compassion, but also our understanding that the pain and despair they are feeling are not signs of weakness or a lack of faith, but of a serious illness. The encouragement we then offer can be especially impactful because it is informed by the knowledge that there are effective treatments for depression. We can help even more by providing them with or directing them to reliable sources of information about treatments.

It's important to understand that even with our words of support and encouraging news about treatment, depressed individuals may find it challenging to obtain the care they need. Tasks that would not have seemed difficult before they became depressed – scheduling an appointment with their doctor, finding a mental health provider who accepts their insurance, arranging transportation to their appointment or finding childcare while they are at their appointment – may seem overwhelming. These are the type of tasks we can assist with, and it may be only because of such assistance that they are able to receive the care they need.

The need for support and encouragement doesn't necessarily end when someone begins treatment. The benefits of both medication and psychotherapy aren't immediate. It can take several weeks to notice a difference. During this period, our expressions of love and support can help depressed individuals stay afloat emotionally and remain committed to their treatment. But they also do much more – they become part of the healing process. I know they were for me. They were powerful reminders that I was not alone and that I was loved and valued – even during my darkest times.

CHAPTER 7

RESOURCES

There are a number of organizations and agencies that have materials and other resources that can be utilized in congregational programs addressing depression and other mental health conditions. One organization I have worked with for several years is the **National Alliance on Mental Illness** (www.nami.org), often referred to as simply "**NAMI**." This organization started as a small group of families in 1979 and now has more than 500 local affiliates. Some affiliates, including NAMI Metropolitan Baltimore, offer an annual mental health conference for faith leaders and collaborate with faith communities on other programs. There are also several programs offered by NAMI that can be of help to individuals and families impacted by depression and other mental health conditions. For example:

> ⇨ NAMI Family-to-Family is a class for families, significant others and friends of people with

mental health conditions. The course is designed to facilitate a better understanding of mental health conditions, increase coping skills and empower participants to become better advocates for their family members.

⇨ NAMI Peer-to-Peer is a class for adults with mental health conditions. The course is designed to encourage growth, healing and recovery among participants.

⇨ NAMI Connection is a support group for people with mental health conditions. Groups meet weekly, every other week or monthly, depending on location.

⇨ NAMI In Our Own Voice offers presentations for the general public to promote awareness of mental health conditions and recovery.

NAMI also has fact sheets that provide information on a number of mental health topics, including:

⇨ Depression
⇨ Bipolar Disorder
⇨ Risk of Suicide
⇨ Self-harm
⇨ Crisis Services
⇨ Medications
⇨ Mental Health Professionals

Mental Health America (www.mhanational.org), founded in 1909, is a community-based nonprofit organization dedicated to addressing the needs of those living with mental illness and promoting the overall mental health of all Americans. The organization, with more than 200 local affiliates in 42 states, offers a variety of materials, online tools, programs and events. On its website, there is information on:

⇨ Co-occurring Disorders and Depression
⇨ Depression in African Americans
⇨ Depression in Teens
⇨ Depression in Older Adults
⇨ Depression in Women
⇨ Dealing With Treatment-Resistant Depression: What To Do When Treatment Doesn't Seem To Work

The **Depression and Bipolar Support Alliance** (www. dbsalliance.org) is a national organization focusing on mood disorders. It offers online and print resources, and has more than 200 affiliate chapters that offer peer-run support groups. The website includes brochures on:

⇨ Finding Peace of Mind: Treatment Strategies for Depression
⇨ Understanding Hospitalization for Mental Health
⇨ DBSA Support Groups: An Important Step on the Road to Wellness
⇨ Suicide Prevention and Mood Disorders
⇨ Helping a Friend or Family Member with Depression or Bipolar Disorder

The **National Institute of Mental Health** (www. nimh.nih.gov) is the lead federal agency for research on mental disorders. NIMH offers brochures and fact sheets on depression and other mental health disorders. These are offered in digital format and are available in English and Spanish. Examples are:

⇨ Depression Basics
⇨ Depression in Women: 5 Things You Should Know
⇨ Men and Depression
⇨ Older Adults and Depression
⇨ Teen Depression

MedlinePlus (www.medlineplus.gov) is an online health information resource for patients and their families and friends. It is a service of the National Library of Medicine, the world's largest medical library, which is part of the National Institutes of Health. Its mission is to present high-quality, relevant health and wellness information that is trusted, easy to understand and free of advertising. It is an excellent resource for information on antidepressant medications. For each medication, you will find answers to important questions, including:

⇨ Why is this medication prescribed?
⇨ How should this medicine be used?
⇨ What special precautions should you follow?
⇨ What special dietary instructions should you follow?
⇨ What side effects can the medication cause?

The **American Psychiatric Association** (www.psychiatry.org) is the main professional organization of psychiatrists in the United States. Its website provides helpful information for patients and families, including a section on depression that discusses:

⇨ Symptoms
⇨ Differences Between Depression and Grief
⇨ Risk Factors for Depression
⇨ Treatments for Depression
⇨ Self-help and Coping

There are also links to related conditions, including:

⇨ Peripartum Depression (previously Postpartum Depression)
⇨ Seasonal Affective Disorder
⇨ Bipolar Disorder

The **American Psychological Association** (www.apa.org) is the largest scientific and professional organization of psychologists in the United States. Its website offers helpful information for patients and families about:

⇨ Depression
⇨ Bipolar Disorder
⇨ Suicide
⇨ Therapy

There also is a link to a fact sheet on depression –
Overcoming Depression: How Psychologists Help with
Depressive Disorders – that can be downloaded.

The **National Suicide Prevention Lifeline** (www.sui-
cidepreventionlifeline.org) provides free and confidential
emotional support to people in suicidal crisis or emotional
distress 24 hours a day, 7 days a week, across the United
States. The Lifeline (1-800-273-8255) is comprised of a
national network of over 150 local crisis centers, combin-
ing custom local care and resources with national stan-
dards and best practices.

Another service available for individuals experiencing
a crisis is the **Crisis Text Line** (www.crisistextline.org).
This is a free service available 24 hours a day, 7 days a
week, throughout the United States. By texting 741741,
individuals are connected with a trained crisis counselor.

Clergy and lay leaders interested in learning how to recognize and respond to mental health crisis situations may
want to consider the **Mental Health First Aid** (www.
mentalhealthfirstaid.org) program. This is an 8-hour
national certification course that teaches lay people how
to recognize the signs and symptoms of an emerging mental health problem or crisis, identify community resources,
and link individuals in need of treatment and support to
the proper resources.

ACKNOWLEDGMENTS

I t would not have been possible to write this book without the love, support and advice of my wife, Kim, my daughter, Graham and my son, Will. They shared many of the experiences I have written about, and they continue to share my commitment to bring the important topic of depression out of the darkness and into the light.

I want to express my appreciation to Sherry Welch and Debbie Hickman for encouraging me to take on this writing project. Having heard me speak a number of times about my experiences with depression, they both insisted that I put these experiences and lessons into print.

I am especially grateful for the valuable editorial assistance I received from Meghan Rossbach, who also offered her friendship and encouragement throughout the writing. Additionally, I want to acknowledge the contributions of Panagis Galiatsatos, Pat Fosarelli and Kate Dunn, each of whom carefully reviewed the manuscript and offered many helpful suggestions.

ABOUT THE AUTHOR

Dan Hale is Special Advisor to the President of Johns Hopkins Bayview Medical Center and Director of the Healthy Community Partnership. He also is an Assistant Professor at the Johns Hopkins University School of Medicine, with appointments in the Department of Psychiatry & Behavioral Sciences and the Division of Geriatric Medicine & Gerontology. Prior to assuming his position at Johns Hopkins Bayview in 2011, Dr. Hale was Professor of Clinical Psychology at Stetson University. A national leader in health ministries, he is the co-author of *Building Healthy Communities through Medical-Religious Partnerships,* published by Johns Hopkins University Press and now in its third edition (2018), and *Healing Bodies and Souls: A Practical Guide for Congregations* (Fortress Press, 2003). In 2016 he was named Mental Health Professional of the Year by NAMI Metropolitan Baltimore, and in 2018 he received the Maryland Foundation for Psychiatry Anti-Stigma Advocacy Prize.